Praise for *The Art & Science of Meditation*

"Whether you are a new or experienced meditator, *The Art & Science of Meditation* is like a wise and experienced companion guiding you through the uncharted terrain of your own heart-mind. Drawing from a vast range of meditation experience, including yogic and Buddhist traditions, Erickson skillfully offers practical and joyful ways to nurture and expand your understanding of meditation."

—Kaveri Patel, DO, family physician and author of *The Voice*

"Lisa Erickson has written the ultimate meditation handbook that is at once deeply engaging, relevant to modern life, practical, and comprehensive. By mapping out a wide range of systems, potential traps, and the full set of meditative stages that may be experienced, she makes even the most advanced stages of meditation accessible and easy to understand. Lisa's book is potent because it will support you immediately and through a lifetime of practice."

—Mu, author of *From Here to Nowhere*

"Lisa Erickson is the wisest of today's meditation guides. In *The Art & Science of Meditation*, she delivers, meeting you right where you are with a myriad of time-proven ways to explore the form of meditation that honors the uniqueness of you. This book is genuinely the most innovative and inter-spiritual resource for meditation I've ever read. I'll be recommending it to all of our students."

—Dr. Janice Lundy, inter-spiritual educator and cofounder of the Spiritual Guidance Training Institute

D0827913

The
Art & Science
of
Meditation

About the Author

Lisa Erickson is an energy worker, writer, and teacher. She has meditated for over thirty years in multiple traditions and is certified in mindfulness meditation instruction, trauma sensitivity, and several healing modalities. She has taught meditation in corporate settings, schools, community centers, rape crises centers, and online. She is also the author of *Chakra Empowerment for Women* and aids women in feminine life transits and sexual trauma healing. Visit her at www.EnlightenedEnergetics.com.

The
Art & Science
of
Meditation

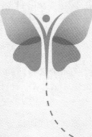

How to Deepen and
Personalize Your Practice

LISA ERICKSON

Llewellyn Publications
Woodbury, Minnesota

FIRST EDITION
First Printing, 2020

Book design by Samantha Penn
Cover design by Kevin Brown
Editing by Laura Kurtz
Illustrations on pages 34, 44, and 108 by Mary Ann Zapalac
    Illustrations on pages 67, 76, 83, 90, 103, 117, 204 and 213 by Llewellyn Art Department

Llewellyn Publications is a registered trademark of Llewellyn Worldwide Ltd.

Library of Congress Cataloging-in-Publication Data (Pending)
Names: Erickson, Lisa, author.
Title: The art & science of meditation : how to deepen and personalize your
    practice / Lisa Erickson.
Other titles: Art and science of meditiation
Description: First edition. | Woodbury, Minnesota : LLewellyn Publications,
    [2020] | Includes index. | Summary: "Beyond beginner level information
    about meditation as a practice, its origins, different styles,
    troubleshooting. Includes figures and exercise"— Provided by publisher.
Identifiers: LCCN 2020018367 (print) | LCCN 2020018368 (ebook) | ISBN
    9780738761398 (paperback) | ISBN 9780738761534 (ebook)
Subjects: LCSH: Meditation—Therapeutic use.
Classification: LCC RC489.M43 E75 2020 (print) | LCC RC489.M43 (ebook) |
    DDC 615.8/52—dc23
LC record available at https://lccn.loc.gov/2020018367
LC ebook record available at https://lccn.loc.gov/2020018368

Llewellyn Publications
A Division of Llewellyn Worldwide Ltd.
2143 Wooddale Drive
Woodbury, MN 55125-2989
www.llewellyn.com

Printed in the United States of America

Other Books by Lisa Erickson

Chakra Empowerment for Women

To all my meditation teachers, past and present.
Thank you for showing me myself.

CONTENTS

Part I
PRACTICE FOR LIFE

Part II
MEDITATION FOR THE
SPIRITUAL SEEKER

Part III
THE PATH

Part IV
MEDITATION IN THE WORLD

PRACTICES

Chapter Six

Chapter Seven

Chapter Eight

Chapter Nine

Chapter Eleven

FIGURES

DISCLAIMER

The information in this book is not intended to be used to diagnose or treat any medical or emotional condition. To address medical or therapeutic issues, please consult a licensed professional.

The author and publisher are not responsible for any conditions that require a licensed professional, and we encourage you to consult a professional if you have any questions about the use or efficacy of the techniques or insights in this book.

All case studies and descriptions of persons have been changed or altered so as to be unrecognizable. Any likeness to actual persons, living or dead, is strictly coincidental.

INTRODUCTION

I remember my first meditation well, more than thirty years ago in a community room on my college's campus. The idea of meditation was entirely new and foreign to me, and I had come to the class at the suggestion of a friend to help with the chronic headaches I had been experiencing. Like many people meditating for the first time, I was shocked to discover how difficult it was to quiet my mind and follow my breath for even a few seconds. As an accomplished student and trained dancer at the time, I took pride in my self-discipline and determination. But here was something I could not simply power my way through. Nevertheless, in the few moments I was able to focus, I touched a peace and stillness I had not known existed within me.

Although I could never have imagined it at the time, that day marked a turning point in my life. In addition to helping with my headaches, which were unquestionably stress-related, that meditation class and the metaphysical questions it triggered for me initiated a deep spiritual search that has continued to this day. Meditation also provided a platform for me to explore energy sensations and intuitions I had often experienced, which led to my eventual studies in energy healing and emotional work (my current field). My appreciation for these different facets of meditation has driven me to both study and teach multiple forms—mindfulness, including certification in order to guide teams in corporate environments; chakra and kundalini meditation as both a spiritual and energy healing foundation for myself and clients; Zen as a complement to martial arts studies; and practices from many different spiritual traditions as part of my spiritual explorations, including my current pathway of Tibetan Buddhism.

I am interested in both what these forms have in common and how they differ, and while I am definitely a believer in committing to a single meditation practice, I also have experienced the value of learning multiple approaches, because doing so has deepened my own understanding and growth. This, more than anything, is what has guided me to write this book—a belief that the world's spiritual, healing, and scientific traditions all have something to offer the contemporary meditator. My primary goal was to help you go deeper into the areas that most intrigue you by bringing some of this information into one book, with many other book references sprinkled throughout. The topics covered are meant to be *useful* to you, whether you are a long-time meditator seeking new inspiration or an occasional practitioner hoping to increase your engagement.

As I worked to compile the topics for this book, a well-loved quote by Zen master Shunryu Suzuki often came to mind: "In the beginner's mind there are many possibilities, but in the expert's there are few."[1] Regardless of the form we practice, in meditation we attempt to discover our natural beginner's mind—open, relaxed, and uncluttered by emotional turmoil or what we think we know. Trapped in the expert's mind, we become resistant to change and new possibilities, often resulting in stress or blocks. But if the beginner's mind is what we seek through meditation, what does it mean to write a book for non-beginners? What information might actually aid someone's meditation practice without contributing to the expert's trap?

It's one of the many conundrums of meditation that its purpose is to lead us inward into our own innate wisdom, yet so many books have been written and so much expert advice offered on how—and how not—to do it. Knowing when to seek this external help and when to let go of it and rely wholly on what arises within yourself is part of the journey of meditation. Whatever

---

1. Shunryu Suzuki, *Zen Mind, Beginner's Mind: Informal Talks on Zen Meditation and Practice*, (Shambhala Press, 2011), 1.

you are looking for, I hope you find it in this book and that it strengthens your inner connection to your own knowing. Take what is useful to you and leave the rest.

How to Use This Book

Meditation truly is both art and science—something highly personal that we create (and continuously recreate) from within ourselves *and* an intricate process with steps we can follow, methods we can employ, and stages we can progress through. In my experience, whatever brings each of us to meditation, we encounter many of the same challenges and questions; in this book, I have sought to offer guidance on these by turning to both classic spiritual texts and contemporary scientific research. I have tried to provide both depth and breadth: depth in terms of diving deep into the wisdom of meditation traditions that are thousands of years old, such as Buddhism and yoga, and breadth by providing information on many different meditation forms and challenges, as well as contemporary research on how meditation affects the mind and body.

This is not a how-to book in the sense of instructions for how to meditate. My assumption is that you already meditate and are looking for ways to modify or enhance your practice. To that end, every chapter includes Practice sections related to the material covered; some are meditation exercises so that you may experiment with other forms. In addition, every chapter ends with a Contemplations section that contains a series of questions you can use to journal with or simply contemplate (hence the name) to personalize the content for yourself. I encourage you to engage with these Practices and Contemplations as tools for exploring the material's application in your own life.

I have tried to keep the book overall relevant to any meditator regardless of faith. It is therefore not an in-depth guide to meditation within any one tradition, although I have turned to Buddhism and yoga for guidance on the stages of meditation in part II, as these two traditions offer the oldest and most comprehensive maps. Of course, if you practice meditation within a particular spiritual tradition, you may also want to consider teachings from within it to aid you with any questions that arise. Here you will hopefully find practical tips based in research or another tradition that aid your practice without contradicting your faith.

You can read this book all the way through or dip in and out, using it as a reference when you encounter specific hurdles or questions. In part I, "Practice for Life," we focus on the various reasons we meditate, cover tips for handling the most common meditation challenges, followed by an overview of scientific research on how different forms of meditation affect the brain. In part II, "Meditation for the Spiritual Seeker," we cover the stages of meditation as described in the most well-known yogic and Buddhist texts on this subject, as well as look at models of spiritual growth from other wisdom traditions. In part III, "The Path," we examine ways for handling subtler meditation challenges, understanding mystic experiences, how to avoid common meditation traps, and how to select or plan a meditation retreat or pilgrimage. In our final section, part IV, "Meditation in the World," we cover the role of a meditation teacher, how gender and social concerns may affect our meditation journey, when and how to share our meditation practice with others in our life, and how to integrate our practice with our daily life.

Books have been a valued resource for me on my path, and indeed entire books have been written on the topics of most of this book's chapters. I have included quotes from many of my favorites throughout this book, as well as including a recommended book list (doubling as my annotated bibliography), in the hopes these will help you to connect with additional resources on the topics that most interest you.

Enjoy the Journey

Regardless of why you have come to this book, I hope most of all that it inspires you. Meditation takes us on journeys both inner and outer. Since that first meditation more than three decades ago, my own practice has been like the river of my life, always carrying me forward and constantly adapting to the changing landscape of my circumstances. Externally, it has brought me to holy places and meditation centers around the world, including the deserts of the U.S. Southwest, the islands of the Caribbean, the temples of Japan, and the monasteries of Bhutan. I have meditated in my car for ten minutes, alone in a mountain cabin for days, in groups of thousands, in a sleep-deprived state with a newborn baby in my arms, and on a cliff with wild bighorn sheep looking on.

Inwardly has been no less of an adventure. Meditation has taken me into every corner of my being, helping me see and face the darkest bits that I might not otherwise have sought to heal or transform. It's triggered profound insight and greatly expanded my capacity for connection and compassion. I've had blissful experiences and unpleasant ones, become elated and become frustrated, had mystic visions and fallen asleep. I've spent a ridiculous amount of time thinking about what I'm going to have for breakfast when I'm done—so it goes with meditation. But what's always pulled me *back* has been that indefinable part of my awareness that can do so—I come back to my breath, my chakra, my visualization, or my mantra—ultimately, back to myself. This thread of awareness is the one constant in the shifting sands of both our inner and outer landscapes, and with a regular meditation practice we are brought back, over and over again, to this richness within us. And so I offer this book not as an expert steeped in expert's mind, but as a fellow human on a journey along with you. I offer it in the spirit of sharing and hope it is of benefit to you.

PART I
PRACTICE FOR LIFE

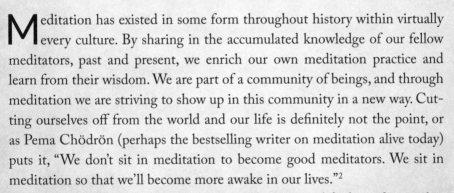

Meditation has existed in some form throughout history within virtually every culture. By sharing in the accumulated knowledge of our fellow meditators, past and present, we enrich our own meditation practice and learn from their wisdom. We are part of a community of beings, and through meditation we are striving to show up in this community in a new way. Cutting ourselves off from the world and our life is definitely not the point, or as Pema Chödrön (perhaps the bestselling writer on meditation alive today) puts it, "We don't sit in meditation to become good meditators. We sit in meditation so that we'll become more awake in our lives."[2]

What it means to you to be more awake in your life depends on what brought you to meditation and why you have continued with it. Perhaps you came to it as a way to relax and manage stress. Perhaps you came to it to improve your concentration, performance, or productivity. Maybe you have issues with anger or depression and hoped meditation would help. Maybe meditation is part of your dedicated personal growth or spiritual path. Or maybe for you, like for me, the role meditation has played in your life has changed over time.

- - - - - - - - - -

2. Pema Chödrön, *When Things Fall Apart: Heart Advice for Difficult Times* (Shambhala Publications, 2000), 21.

In this first part of the book, chapter 1 begins with an exploration of the different reasons people meditate as well as its purposes and benefits as a platform for you to better define for yourself why you practice and what you hope to gain (or lose!). In chapter 2 we will cover tips for handling the most common challenges to meditating, including establishing or increasing routine, drowsiness, busyness, physical pain, and life challenges. Chapter 3 will cover some of the most recent scientific research into meditation and how this might inform your own practice. The Practices and Contemplations in each chapter will help you to integrate the material and utilize it to deepen your own practice for life.

ONE

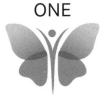

WHY DO YOU PRACTICE?

Before we can dive into the *why*, we need to define the *what*. In the West, meditation has become a blanket term used to describe many different contemplative practices. Specific traditions often have strong opinions on what is or is not meditation, which can become confusing to someone not familiar with the traditions' larger context. In this book we'll cast a wide net but focus on specific forms when discussing benefits and challenges. In general, we'll consider all of the following to fall under the meditation tent:

- Focus on the breath or counting breaths
- Mindfulness: present non-judgmental awareness of feelings and thoughts
- Mantra, seed syllable, or chanting practice
- Focus on sound or sacred music designed for meditative purposes
- Visualization, including of scenes, deities, mandalas, or yantras
- Contemplative energy practices involving chakras or kundalini cultivation
- Compassion or healing practices involving the sending or receiving of intentions and energies
- Contemplation of sacred phrases, texts, or questions

- Contemplation of God, Goddess, Source, or any higher power/law
- Insight or inquiry practices centered on turning the mind inward
- Objectless, or resting, meditation—in which there is no object of focus

These are very disparate forms of meditation, and at first glance it may be hard to see what binds them together. Some can be done either moving or sitting, with eyes open or closed, while others require a particular posture and setting. Some are very active and effortful, i.e., constructing visualizations in the mind or actively inquiring into its contents. Others orient around *releasing* effort—relaxing into the present moment, a higher power, or awareness itself. Some meditation forms are very physical: generating sounds in the case of chanting, focusing on the rise and fall of the belly while breathing, concentrating on a physical location in the case of chakras, and so on. Still others seem to disengage from the body and occur primarily on the mental plane—contemplating a text or question or directing healing thoughts towards others.

Regardless of these differences, we have one common experience when actually engaged in any of these meditation forms, especially in the initial stages—pulling our attention *back* over and over (and over!) again. Whether we are bringing our attention back to our breath, our body, a visual, a chant, a phrase, or resting, our experience is one of having wandered away from our intended focus, and then returning to it through pulling our attention back. This basic movement—away and back, away and back—defines much of our time in meditation.

What pulls us away, what it means to "come back," and what underlies both is defined differently within various traditions and comprises a large amount of what's been written about meditation over the centuries. We will investigate these questions in future chapters; but on a more general level, exploring the word *practice* provides deeper insight into what different meditation forms have in common. No matter what form we engage in, we are *practicing* pulling our attention back. The act of returning to our meditation, and indeed, some would say to our very selves, is what defines the experience. With time, we may settle into a level of awareness in which this movement away and back is itself experienced as waves within a vaster expanse, but then we may move in and out of this awareness. Anchoring in that which never moves and within which all other movement occurs (some might call it awareness of awareness, others might call it God, Source, or Spirit) is the essence of spiritual meditation. Regardless of the conceptual framework, returning or pulling our attention back is what we practice when we sit.

What are we practicing *for*? To relate to our mind and reality differently. By default, the mind runs wherever it likes, ruled by emotions and our immediate reactions to our experiences. Like I was, first time meditators are usually astonished and often dismayed to discover how unruly the mind actually is. In meditation, we practice something other than this. Just as a dancer or athlete must practice to change the manner in which their bodies move, we practice to change how our mind conducts itself. At first, we attempt to tame or quiet its unruliness—we are practicing mental calmness—and it yields many benefits. We may also practice many other things depending on the form of meditation we engage in—attentiveness, compassion, inquisitiveness, self-awareness, energy activation, positivity, connection with God or Source—but whatever we practice is different from our default. Our formal sitting meditation is a protected time for us to *practice living differently*.

So, what are *you* practicing, and why? What is your motivation? Engaging with these questions can help you refine your meditation practice as well as reinspire it. We are often told not to judge our meditations or think in terms of goals because we would then be practicing self-criticism and achievement, two things most of us already practice quite frequently off the meditation cushion. However, contemplating and refining our *motivation* as opposed to goals can be quite helpful to us. The concept of motivation and its related aspect, intention, play a big role in virtually every meditation tradition.

The next few sections cover some of the most common motivations for meditating along with which meditation forms are associated with each. More in-depth information related to all of these appear in later chapters, but these initial sections may help you distinguish the various forms of meditation available as well as their commonalities and differences. As you read through these sections, contemplate what brought *you* to meditation. Have your needs changed?

Relaxation and Resilience

Meditation is now synonymous with *relaxation* in the minds of many—I am often met with "Oh, how relaxing!" when I mention I am going on a meditation retreat (if they only knew!). This is unfortunate in some ways, because when first-time meditators confront their monkey minds and do not initially feel relaxed, they sometimes discount meditation's benefits and don't try again. The truth, as you've probably experienced yourself, is a little more complicated. Sure, there are meditation forms that are designed specifically to induce a relaxation response in our body and forms that help us disconnect from stress-inducing thoughts, *but* meditation is rarely an instantaneous antidote to our stress.

Nevertheless, relaxation and stress management are the primary motivation for many meditators, and meditating for these reasons can have great health benefits. Stress contributes to dozens of diseases; reversing its harmful impact on our body prevents some of these from taking hold and speeds our recovery from others. In various research over the past forty years, meditation has been linked to lowering blood pressure, countering insomnia, decreasing headache frequency, and easing irritable bowel syndrome—all maladies linked to stress.

However, more research is still needed to determine exactly which meditation forms work for this purpose, for whom, and in what circumstances. For example, a recent meta-analysis of past studies that had linked meditation to lowered blood pressure yielded mixed results: some of the studies' methodologies did not meet scientific standards, while others were difficult to cross-analyze because of variations in the length of time individuals were asked to meditate, the level of training and support they received, or the level of hypertension they were experiencing before they began the study.[3]

The discrepancy of findings does not invalidate the idea that meditation contributes to lowering blood pressure or stress management in general, but it does indicate that we need to be careful about the medical claims made about meditation. What studies *have* consistently borne out is that partici-

- - - - - - - - - - - -

3. Lu Shi, et al., "Meditation and Blood Pressure: A Meta-Analysis," *Journal of Hypertension* 35, no. 4 (April 2017): 696–706, https://journals.lww.com/jhypertension/Abstract/2017/04000/Meditation_and_blood_pressure___a_meta_analysis_of.5.aspx.

pants self-report a different relationship to their feelings of stress and anxiety after meditating regularly. The most robust research in this area revolves around Mindfulness-Based Stress Reduction, or MBSR, developed by Dr. Jon Kabat-Zinn in the 1970s as a secularized form of Buddhist-based mindfulness meditation. Participants are most likely to report this shifted relationship to their own stress and anxiety when they engage in regular MBSR practice, usually about thirty minutes a day for an eight-week period.[4]

The research on MBSR and related practices has shifted the discussion about meditation for stress from *relaxation* to *resilience*. Relaxation is a specific neuro-physical state characterized by lowered levels of stress hormones, such as adrenaline and cortisol, in our body and increased production of "relaxation" endorphins. While some forms of meditation do appear to successfully induce this relaxation response in our body while we are meditating, it doesn't always carry over into stressful situations during our day. However, the changed relationship to stressful and anxious thoughts and feelings that mindfulness meditation generates *does* appear to carry over into daily life in the form of greater *resilience* overall when we are experiencing a stressful situation. Resilience is defined as our ability to cope with stress or a crisis situation and bounce back from any harmful effects. Recent research indicates that brain changes in longer term meditators actually builds this kind of resilience on a neurological level.[5]

We come back to the question of what you are practicing when you sit down to meditate—are you practicing relaxing, or are you practicing letting go of your attachment to thoughts and emotions as they arise? Both will benefit you and help you lower your average stress point, but only practicing relaxation may not translate to the ability to better handle a work deadline, argument with your spouse, financial crisis, or any other stressful situation. For it to benefit you in these situations, your meditation needs to be practice for recognizing triggered emotions or thoughts as they arise and letting them go. This means that forms designed to induce altered states, visions, or

- - - - - - - - - - - -

4. Sue McGreevey, "Eight Weeks to a Better Brain," The Harvard Gazette, January 21, 2011, https://news.harvard.edu/gazette/story/2011/01/eight-weeks-to-a-better-brain/.

5. Julieta Galante, et al., "A mindfulness-based intervention to increase resilience to stress in university students," *Lancet Public Health* (Dec 2017): 72-81, https://www.thelancet.com/journals/lanpub/article/PIIS2468-2667(17)30231-1/fulltext.

in some cases even mantras that are deeply centering and relaxing (inducing the body's relaxation response), however good they may feel in the moment, may not always translate into increased resilience and stress management benefits.

A student in one of my corporate mindfulness classes discovered this difference of practice for herself. Diane worked in a high-stress technology environment with frequent deadlines. She had meditated for many years but was frustrated by how little it seemed to help her when under stress. When facing a deadline, she became increasingly short-tempered and often experienced insomnia. As we talked more about her practice, it was clear that Diane had become very adept at sitting down and relaxing through the mantra-based practice she'd had for years, and she often experienced what she considered to be spiritual energies. She experienced meditation as a kind of temporary medicine: she always felt better afterwards, but it didn't seem to help her when circumstances would trigger her stress response. As we talked, Diane decided to experiment changing her practice up with a mindfulness practice.

When I checked in with Diane several months later, she felt her experiment had been a great success. She practiced a bit of both forms of meditation daily, as she felt they both benefited her in different ways. Practicing breath-based mindfulness, in which she simply observed arising thoughts and emotions and pulled her mind back to her breath, had greatly increased her ability to notice tension in her body as it was arising and let it go in the moment. Her mantra practice continued to provide her connection to spiritual energies she felt she otherwise would not have access to. Furthermore, she believed the two practices together had helped her integrate her meditation more deeply into her daily life.

This theme of integration is one we will return to again and again because it is central to the idea that in meditation we are practicing for our real lives, *not* disengaging. Of course, some forms of meditation are meant to connect us to metaphysical levels of reality we may not become aware of any other way; but for meditation to benefit us in our daily lives, we need to make a connection between those experiences and how we feel when we are walking around interacting in the world. We otherwise run the risk of our practice becoming the foundation for spiritual bypassing or disassociation, two potential meditation traps covered in chapter 8.

Practicing a new relationship to your thoughts and emotions is key to stress management and developing true resilience, which is actually more important in the long run than being able to sit down and instantly relax (though that's always great too!). We will talk more about how a changed relationship to thoughts and emotions reflects as actual physical brain changes amongst meditators in chapter 3.

Practice
- - - - - - - - - - -
MINDFULNESS OF BREATH

If you do not already practice mindfulness meditation, here is a simple breath-based practice to explore it with.

- Settle into an alert and comfortable meditation posture.
- Bring your awareness to the sensation of either your belly rising and falling as you breathe, or the feeling of the air moving in and out of your nose or mouth with each inhale and exhale. (The choice of focal point is yours.)
- Stay present with the sensations associated with breathing at your focal point—the expansion and deflation of your belly, or the warmth of your breath on the skin above your lip. Allow yourself to be inquisitive and notice as much as you can about these sensations.
- As with all forms of meditation, simply pull your mind back to these sensations whenever your mind wanders.

The difference between this and object-based forms of meditation (focusing on a mantra, visual, chakra, or another anchor) is that the emphasis is on staying fully present with the sensation and noticing its qualities and shifts without judgment. Most object-based forms are concentration-based, in which the emphasis is on merging with the object in some way. It is covered in chapter 4.

Mental Wellness and Personal Growth

Because of its power to help us change our relationship to our thoughts and emotions, many mental health practitioners have adopted MBSR and related practices and use them with patients. Studies have shown mindfulness meditation in particular can be a valuable part of treatment for depression, chronic anxiety and trauma.[6] Therapists, addiction counselors in rehab centers, nurses in hospices, school counselors, and many other professionals use it. Indeed, "mindfulness" within these contexts has almost become commonplace, so much so that some worry these practices are becoming too watered down or that overmarketing is undermining their value.[7]

Whatever the method, if you are using meditation as part of treatment for addiction, depression, trauma, or another diagnosed mental health condition, it's always best if done under the guidance of a qualified teacher and/or mental health professional. Sometimes within practice troubling emotions or thoughts can arise; as our usually busy mind settles, aspects of our psyche that we may have repressed or neglected tend to surface. While in the longer term these experiences may be a necessary part of our healing, many individuals need support to process whatever has been repressed or neglected in a healthy way. This is particularly important if you have experienced any form of trauma in your life. (Trauma sensitivity is covered in more depth in chapter 3.)

Many individuals who are or have been in therapeutic treatment also turn to other kinds of healers, spiritual guides, or intuitives for complementary treatment; in fact, there are many other meditation modalities that may

- - - - - - - - - - - -

6. Tamara A. Russell and Gerson Siegmund, "What and who? Mindfulness in the mental health setting," *BJPsych Bulletin* 40, December 2016, 333-340, https://www.cambridge.org/core/journals/bjpsych-bulletin/article/what-and-who-mindfulness-in-the-mental-health-setting/3779267983563980FC1E31781AD3A694.

7. Jon Kabat-Zinn, "Too Early to Tell: The Potential Impact and Challenges—Ethical and Otherwise—Inherent in the Mainstreaming of Dharma in an Increasingly Dystopian World," *Mindfulness Journal,* October 2017, 1125–1135, https://link.springer.com/article/10.1007/s12671-017-0758-2.

be helpful although there is less research available to validate their effectiveness. Here are some other meditation practices that are commonly used in psychological therapy settings:

- Within traditions that work with the subtle (or energy) body, problematic emotional patterns are viewed as part of blocks or dysfunctional energies that can be released and transformed through energy-based meditation practices.
- Mantras and chakra (energy center) techniques are taught to function partly on a vibrational level, shifting a meditator's state of awareness in a way that leads to permanent change.
- Mandala meditations and visualizations are part of several traditions; psychoanalyst Carl Jung (and many subsequent Jungian psychologists) studied them as a means for balancing and integrating disparate aspects of the psyche.
- Visual meditation forms, including guided imagery methods, are used as a means of dialoging with subtle layers of the psyche.

The truth is if we engage in a dedicated meditation practice, it's inevitable we will be working psychologically at some point. As we saw with stress management, the most profound shifts occur as we change our relationship to our thoughts and emotions, and while mindfulness practice can help us to improve our ability to notice these in the moment, deeper change usually requires looking at patterns in our thoughts and emotions, as well as their underlying roots. We might do this through talk therapy, emotional/energy modalities, or a combination of the two. If we come to meditation for spiritual reasons (the next motivation covered), we also will usually be called to work at a psychological level. In every spiritual tradition that employs meditation, spiritual realization or connection requires releasing or cutting through levels of the psyche that block us from recognizing our inherent spirit or natural radiance.

In other words, whether you have viewed it as such or not, meditation involves a potentially a deeply psychologically transformative process. Often transformation happens without us fully realizing its scope, something that struck me while visiting with a college friend whom I had not seen in almost two decades. While I am aware of many of the ways in which meditation has benefited my life, she asked me if I still experienced the strong mood swings and sleep disturbances I had often experienced in college (along with the headaches). At first, I could not even remember what she was talking about until she reminded me of some of the occurrences. I realized these episodes had entirely disappeared from my life in the first few years after college when I began meditating daily. Although meditation has not been a panacea for my life, a certain heaviness I used to experience regularly as a young adult left me permanently, and I feel strongly it is linked to my meditation practice. I have heard many such stories over the years, including very different kinds of transformations: individuals whose food preferences entirely changed in the first few years of regular practice, or for whom previously unknown artistic talents surfaced seemingly out of the blue. We are complex, layered beings; meditation allows us to touch and release parts of ourselves we might otherwise never reach.

It is this power for aiding transformation that has brought meditation into many personal development programs. The Human Potential Movement of the 1960s incorporated meditation modalities from primarily Eastern spiritual sources that eventually became the foundation for the modern self-help industry. Meditation is incorporated into programs from weight loss to personal improvement, financial gain to relationship help. Although the methods vary, in many cases the emphasis is on meditation as a means of changing limiting or harmful thought patterns—often cultivating positive emotions or replacing thought patterns through visualization or repeating affirmations.

In some ways, these methodologies are the opposite of mindfulness practice. Rather than being with whatever is present, in these meditation forms we cultivate particular thoughts, emotions, energies, or visuals we wish to experience in greater quantities. We practice new mental and emotional patterns and thus strengthen our capacity to experience them outside of meditation. This form of practice also has science behind it in the form of relatively recent breakthroughs in the study of neuroplasticity—the ability of our brain to change through learning and conscious mental activity. In other words, what we choose to think now can actually change our neuropathways and influence what thoughts will arise later. Neuroplasticity is covered in more depth in chapter 3.

For now, if you came to meditation for help with mental health issues, make sure you are receiving the support you need. If you came to it for personal transformation, think about whether what you are practicing in meditation is cultivating the change you seek. If you did not come to meditation for either of these reasons, think about how your practice may need to deepen to a psychological level in order for you to truly get what you seek from it.

Spiritual Realization

While the forms of meditation discussed so far are primarily secular, history shows that meditation developed within spiritual traditions around the world. Every major world religion has included some form of meditation, and the vast amount of material on meditation has come from these sources. Regardless of whether or not your own motivation for meditating is spiritual, you may find much in this material that is helpful to you, and we will spend three chapters (the entirety of part II) on spiritual models for the stages of meditation.

To really get a sense of the spiritual foundation of meditation, consider these various forms:

- In Buddhism, observing and stilling the mind are the key to recognizing the transience of all thoughts and emotions, opening the doorway to realizing our innate enlightened mind.
- In the yogic branches of Hinduism and Vedanta, meditating is the core practice for merging the mind with the energies operating beneath the physical world through which the mind can ultimately merge with the source of these energies itself. Meditation is considered part of yoga practice: *yoga* means "union," and meditation is considered the primary method for merging our awareness with the divine.
- In Kabbalah (often called Jewish mysticism), a form of meditation called *hitbonenut*, which involves contemplating a concept or light itself, is used to attain true, meta-intellectual knowledge.

- Eastern Orthodox Christianity incorporates the *hesychasm,* or Jesus prayer, performed in a meditative, chanting fashion, in order to connect with the heart of faith.

- Roman Catholicism includes contemplative practices such as the rosary for lay people, and many silent contemplative practices for monastic initiates. St. Teresa of Avila was one of several Catholic mystics who wrote on the benefits of "mental prayer," and Ignatius Loyola taught a form of Jesuit meditation.

- At Quaker meetings, participants sit in silence, waiting for the "inner light" to inspire someone to speak.

- The Sufis within Islam incorporate both energy center and devotional meditation to merge with the beloved divine responsible for life itself. Sufism has many branches and corresponding meditation techniques, but most are centered on love meditations.

- Taoism is the ancient Chinese mystic religious tradition and philosophy focused on balance and the interacting forces of yin/yang, passive/aggressive, masculine/feminine, and creating/receiving. Tai chi is often considered a form of moving Taoist meditation, and sitting Taoist meditation focuses on similar themes of balance and flow.

- The Baha'i faith, founded in nineteenth-century Persia, incorporates meditation as a means to experience spiritual unity with all humankind and the common themes of all world religions.

- Many indigenous cultures incorporate contemplative methods into their spirituality, including as healing practices, within coming of age rituals, and as a means for seeking divine guidance.

While each of these traditions have their own theology, a common theme is that meditation provides a means for connecting with a level of awareness, spirit, or spiritual forces that we normally either don't notice or can't comprehend. Our everyday mind is so full of chatter, memories, perceptions, and desires that we block out a connection to the divine or Source. Through meditation, we quiet all of this and discover something vaster than our usual selves. Depending on the tradition, this vastness is seen as our doorway to a deeper understanding of reality, true compassion for others, and union with the sacred laws that define our universe. We come to know ourselves as part of something greater.

What is fascinating to me is how meditators from different traditions throughout history have described such similar spiritual experiences. Infinite light, timelessness, spaciousness, and unconditional love have been described by practitioners from virtually every contemplative tradition. Their interpretations of these experiences may differ after they emerge from meditation, and any beings or deities envisioned may conform to their own specific background; but on a more abstract level, more is the same than different. Some neuroscientists have begun to explore the roots of this as well, which will be covered briefly in chapter 3, and it is these commonalities that forms the basis for my own belief that learning about the stages of meditation as defined in multiple spiritual traditions—as we will do in part II of this book—can benefit anyone of any faith. It is also part of what has fueled my studies in the subtle or energy body, as I view energy practices as spiritual technology that any meditator is in fact engaging with while practicing, whether consciously or not. Some of these principles are covered in later chapters as well.

If your meditation is part of a particular spiritual tradition, then of course you will want to consider everything you read here within the context of your own beliefs. Or perhaps you came to meditation as a secular practice, but your experience with it has triggered questioning that is leading you towards spiritual explorations. Either way, in this regard, meditation is the *experiential* arm of spirituality rather than the *theoretical*. On a spiritual level, meditation is where we explore and realize spirit directly, beyond theology, philosophy, or metaphysics, all of which can quickly become intellectual gymnastics. To me, this is what makes meditation ultimately empowering and even radical—you can use it decide for yourself what you believe.

Contemplations

As we've seen, the field of meditation is vast! You are engaged in a universal process that has been discovered, developed, and refined by many individuals around the world in different times and places for different purposes. So now let's focus on *your* journey; before moving on, take a moment to contemplate the following questions for yourself:

- What initially brought you to meditation? What form did you begin with?

- Were your initial goals realized? Have you experimented with other meditation forms?

- What is your current motivation? Has it changed?

- Have you had experiences in meditation you consider spiritual? How do you interpret them?

- What has been the most empowering aspect of meditation for you? What has been the most challenging?

- What has brought you to this book? What are you hoping to learn or get help with?

Whether your motivation for meditating is to relax, improve your health, change your life, achieve enlightenment, or experience the divine, actual practice is key. Meditation is something you *do*, not just study. Whatever form you engage in, while you meditate you are practicing something different from your usual way of being, and we all encounter similar challenges to practice. Before we dive deeper into how meditation affects the brain, let's look in chapter 2 at some of these common challenges and advice for handling them.

TWO

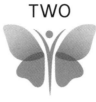

COMMON CHALLENGES

If you have an established meditation practice, you may already have strategies for dealing with the challenges outlined in this chapter—stabilizing a meditation routine, drowsiness, mental busyness, physical pain, illness, and life events that disrupt your practice. These are all challenges that almost every beginning meditator struggles with. But it's also quite common for these to arise throughout our meditation lifetime as our body and circumstances change. You may not have experienced physical pain while meditating when younger, but now you're in your fifties and your hips are starting to object. You may have come to an acceptance and understanding about bouts of drowsiness or excessive mental activity in your meditation and not consider it a challenge, but then a life event leaves you reeling and suddenly your mind is so busy that you need to approach your practice differently. I have experienced both situations myself, and so wanted to include this chapter. We will discuss subtler challenges in chapters 7 and 8—working with emotions and mental disturbances, as well as how to process mystic or energetic experiences. But I find that the challenges outlined in this chapter tend to recur, and it's always worth revisiting ideas for refreshing your approach to them.

Stabilizing or Upping Your Routine

Often the biggest challenge to practice is stabilizing a regular routine. While meditating here and there may be rewarding, regularity is key to experiencing almost any of the known benefits. Fortunately, the last decade's worth of research into how we can support ourselves in the development of a new habit has provided much insight. You can also apply these tips to increasing the frequency or length of your meditation or to any change in your meditation routine you would like to make.

One of the most important findings is on the length of time it takes to develop a new daily habit from a neurological perspective, or the point at which it becomes automatic to our brain and we do not need to employ so much effort. While there is no set length of time that works for everyone and every habit, research indicates that two months is the average.[8] If you aren't meditating daily but would like to, doing so for about two months will vastly increase your chances of continuing to do so for the rest of your life. If you are not interested in meditating daily but would like to increase the frequency and regularity of your meditations, you can adjust this number proportionally: two months of meditation is about sixty days' worth, so if you want to meditate three times a week, allow yourself twenty weeks (also sixty days' worth) to establish this as a habit.

Setting realistic goals is key to your success. If you've been meditating once a week for twenty minutes, setting a goal of meditating two hours daily is not your best chance at success. Really look at your life, your motivation for meditating, and your current meditation practice, and think about a realistic increase in regularity and/or length of meditation time that you believe would benefit you. Breaking your goal down into smaller goals is often helpful too—if your eventual goal is to meditate every day but you are currently meditating a couple of times a month, shoot for three times a week as a start, and reassess as you make progress.

When in a routine-building or routine-increasing phase, there are many things you can do to improve your chances of sticking with your plan. The

--- --- --- --- --- --- ---

8. Phillippa Lally, et al., "How are habits formed: Modelling habit formation in the real world," *European Journal of Social Psychology* 40, October 2010, 998–1009, https://onlinelibrary .wiley.com/doi/abs/10.1002/ejsp.674.

most important is to focus on developing prompts for your brain linked to meditation. The easiest way to do this is to meditate at the same time, and in the same place, every day, and to always precede your meditation with the same activities. For example, perhaps you get up, have a cup of coffee or tea, and sit right down to meditate. Perhaps you like to shower, exercise, or eat a light breakfast as well first. Whatever it is, define a routine and stick to it. Don't vary the order from day to day. On the days you have decided are your "meditation days," keep to your routine. Over time, this regularity is part of what prompts your brain to expect meditation; that is, this consistency is what forms a habit on the actual neurological level.

Building prompts into your meditation location is key too. Create an environment where you can place items related to your meditation motivation and intentions around you. Perhaps these are relaxing or sacred pictures, a candle, incense, or flowers. In general, you don't want pictures of you and your loved ones because you are trying to prompt your mind to take a break from its usual focus. Use the same chair or cushion each day, or consider pampering yourself with a new blanket or back pillow that will only be used in your meditation. Incorporate your favorite colors. If you can't dedicate a specific space to meditation full time, consider creating a mobile box that contains some of these items you can take out each day when you meditate. Again, the key is creating prompts for your brain.

Another key finding of habit development research is related to what's known as the reward cycle.[9] Our brain is hardwired to respond to reward, and in fact the promise of reward can speed the development of a habit faster than almost anything else. When we experience pleasure—whether triggered by a favorite food, shopping for clothes, or hearing a favorite song—our body releases endorphins. When this is regularly preceded by another activity, our brain begins to link the two, experiencing the latter as a reward for the prior. Of course, the main "rewards" of meditation are abstract and longer term—stress management, resilience, personal growth, spiritual realization. When in a habit-forming phase, consider providing yourself with a

- - - - - - - - - - - -

9. Allison Phillips, et al., "Intrinsic rewards predict exercise via behavioral intentions for initiators but via habit strength for maintainers," *Sport, Exercise, and Performance Psychology* 5, November 2016, 352–364, https://psycnet.apa.org/doiLanding?doi=10.1037%2Fspy0000071.

more tangible and consistent post-meditation treat. It may seem paradoxical to reward yourself with a piece of chocolate or foot rub after meditating each day, but the anticipation of this treat will help your brain form a connection; and once it has, you can forgo the reward. You are training your brain!

In the contemporary world, an important part of creating your routine around meditation is taking an honest look at your relationship to the screens in your life, whether this means your smartphone, tablet, computer, or television. As we have come to accept the presence of screens, the 24/7 access to them and all they connect us with in our lives, research shows that we have actually lost our ability to disconnect from them. Many of us actually experience the reward cycle of our brains when we see "likes" on our social media posts, view responses to emails and texts, or click on online news articles that confirm our values or point of view.[10] It can be very difficult to disengage from this cycle for any length of time, which means that for your meditation routine to stick, you may have to be brutally honest and define strict rules for yourself regarding this, i.e., not looking at your phone before meditating each day, or not allowing it (or any screens) near you during meditation.

One exception to eliminating screens involves apps that include guided meditations, meditation music or soundscapes, and timers. For some people, apps that assist in meditation are a valuable resource and can be quite motivating for their practice. Your experience with using these apps may be a sort of reward in and of itself wherein they fuel your practice rather than distract from it. These apps can be wonderful for integrating the prevalence of technology into a practice, supporting integration with daily life. That said, the key is in the details: When using such apps, are you really able to let go of everything else on your phone or device? If even the presence of your phone nearby triggers constant thoughts of "I wonder if so-and-so responded to my text," the cons of the distraction may outweigh the pros of the app. As with everything related to meditation, self-honesty is crucial.

One piece of good news that has come out of habit development research is that it's okay to miss a day here and there. If you are trying to establish a daily practice, missing a few days over the course of two months doesn't seem

- - - - - - - - - - - -

10. Lauren Sherman, et al, "What the brain 'Likes': neural correlates of providing feedback on social media," *Social Cognitive and Affective Neuroscience* 13, July 2018, 699–707, https://doi.org/10.1093/scan/nsy051.

to lengthen the time it takes to develop it as a habit. However, if you go two or more days in a row, that does have an impact. It's important that when you do miss a day or goal, you return to your routine as quickly as possible.

Practice

ESTABLISHING A NEW MEDITATION HABIT

If one of your meditation challenges is lack of regularity or you'd like to increase your routine, incorporate these findings from habit development research to help you:

- Determine a realistic goal. Break a larger goal into smaller, shorter-term goals.
- Create prompts for your brain through an established routine.
- Create prompts by establishing a dedicated meditation space (or mobile box).
- Offer yourself an immediate post-meditation reward, at least during the habit-forming or habit-changing phase.
- Carefully assess your screen use and location during meditation.

Busy vs. Drowsy Mind

One oft-used metaphor I like for meditation is that of tuning a guitar string. If the string is too tight it might snap, but it won't make a sound if it is too loose. In meditation, if our mind is too tense, it often becomes busy and we lose our focus, but if it is too loose, we become spacey or drowsy. Meditation practice is the process of tuning and finding the middle ground—a clear and alert yet calm and focused state. It is often also about finding a balance between trying too hard, becoming too forced or effortful, and being too relaxed—not directing our mind at all in the name of surrendering to something greater but actually just spacing out.

Most meditation instruction includes guidance on how to navigate between these two aspects of mind. Bhante Gunaratana, author of the classic

Mindfulness in Plain English, calls them the "thinking mind" and the "sinking mind." A thinking mind is a busy mind, wherein our thoughts bounce from thought to thought in a seemingly endless train of mental activity. The sinking mind is its opposite, describing when we fall into a kind of stupor that might manifest as drowsiness, but often doesn't actually become physical fatigue. Gunaratana describes it like this:

> [S]inking denotes any dimming of awareness. At its best, it is sort of a mental vacuum in which there is no thought, no observation of the breath, no awareness of anything. It is a gap, a formless mental gray area rather like a dreamless sleep.[11]

It's easy to mistake sinking mind for relaxation or detachment; some people develop the idea that meditation should be an emotionless, sensory-deprived state. In fact, ideally in meditation we cultivate a clear, alert, calm awareness. Instead of *manufacturing* this as a state, we *discover* it through meditating. On the other hand, it's also common to become fixated on "no thought" as the goal of meditation, the antithesis of thinking mind. This kind of fixation can cause us to artificially shut down our thought activity and force a mental blank wall that is also not a clear, alert, calm awareness.

The classics mention *concentration* and *focus* as the tools to address a busy mind—pulling our mind back from distractions repeatedly to quiet our primary mental activity. Whatever is our intended object of meditation, be it our breath, a chakra, a visualization, a mantra, or awareness itself, we continuously pull our mind back to this focal point, attempting to do so without judgment. Although it is sometimes useful to contemplate the nature of our distractions (e.g., major themes and duration) after giving this only brief attention, we pull our mind back to our focal point.

For a drowsy or spacey mind, *curiosity* is our primary helpmate. We can examine the nature of the drowsiness itself, look at its qualities as a sensation, and compare it with alertness. We can also contemplate how it impacts our body, or emotions. Doing this helps us pull back from the dimness of

---

11. Bhante Henepola Gunaratana, *Mindfulness in Plain English: 20th Anniversary Edition,* (Wisdom Publications, 2011), 70.

this state into an alert and inquisitive mode. From here, we can return to our point of focus, whether it is our breath or something else. If drowsiness or spaceyness are a recurrent problem, it's sometimes helpful to do more active meditations for a time (e.g., adding counting to a breath meditation, rotating through the chakras in a chakra meditation, or focusing on our senses mindfully—what we hear, smell, and so on) in order to keep ourselves in an alert, inquisitive state.

Most strategies for dealing with a busy or drowsy mind are variations on these basic approaches. For busyness, slow down mental activity through greater stability, and for drowsiness/spaceyness increase activity in a guided way. Here are some other ways to work with these approaches:

- **The breath.** In general, elongating your exhales will trigger relaxation and help you slow your thoughts, while elongating your inhales will stimulate your body and increase your alertness. If you find yourself struggling with a busy mind, try breathing in on a 4 count and out on a 6 count for several breaths, and/or hold at the bottom of your exhale for a second or two. For a drowsy or spacey mind, reverse this: inhale for 6 to 8 counts while exhaling in 4, and/or briefly hold at the top of your inhalation.

- **The body.** Focusing on your lower body, and in particular your seat and connection to the floor or earth, will help you to ground and stabilize an excessively busy mind. Focusing on the rise and fall of your belly as you breathe can also have this effect. Bringing your awareness upward, to the feel of your breath as it moves in and out of your nose, or to the sensations in your face will help to increase your alertness if feeling drowsy or spacey.

- **Lower vs. upper chakras.** If you are familiar with the chakras and/or engaged in chakra meditation, focus for a time on your root chakra focal point at the base of your tailbone if your mind is very busy, or on your third eye if you are drowsy.

- **Stretch and balance.** If you are really caught up in either intense busyness or drowsiness, take a break to work with your body. Stretch upward and take deep breaths to increase alertness. To decrease mental activity and increase your concentration, focus on balancing on one leg or a balancing yoga posture.

- **Body sequencing.** For a busy mind, imagine relaxing one body part at a time from your head down; for a drowsy mind, imagine waking up piece by piece from your feet upward.

- **Inquisitiveness.** Be curious about what you are experiencing. Although inquisitiveness is often recommended for addressing a drowsy mind, it can also be helpful for a thinking, active one. Seek where in your mind the thoughts are arising from, or where in your body the drowsiness seems to dominate. Are there emotions involved in either? If so, where are they in your body?

- **Affirmations.** Say a few affirmations out loud that counter what you are feeling: "I am calm and my mind is quiet" if feeling overly active, or "I am alert and energetic" if feeling drowsy, or "I am fully present and engaged" if spacey.

- **Label and move on.** Say "thinking" when you pull back from the busy mind state and then let it go. Say "sinking" when you catch yourself dozing off or spacing out and move on.

Whatever tuning method you use, consider it a brief interlude, and come back to the core method of your meditation afterwards. Your ability to notice your state of awareness, select a tool to address it, and pull your mind back *is* your meditation—the activity of tuning—and it yields many benefits.

If you find that you consistently struggle with one or the other—thinking/busy or sinking/drowsy/spacey mind—you may want to consider how this pattern reflects your mind state outside of meditation. When under stress or experiencing difficulty, do you become frenetic and worry constantly, spinning in anxious thoughts of what might occur or how you can prevent it? Or do you tune out, seek escape, and disconnect from the present moment and those who care about you? Often challenges in meditation reflect larger coping strategies (some of which may be unhealthy), so we could benefit from working to understand and change them outside of meditation through counseling or personal development programs. This is where that intersection between meditation and psychological work takes place.

If you experience the same issue consistently in your meditation, you may also want to look at external factors. A colleague once asked me how she could keep from falling asleep in meditation, telling me she had tried all of the suggestions above. As we spoke, I finally thought to ask her how much sleep she was getting nightly, to which she responded, "Oh, I only have time for three to four hours most nights." Not really a mystery why she was falling asleep! While for some people meditation does become more rejuvenating than sleep, that takes time, and the body has certain needs that must be addressed. Similarly, too much caffeine or media exposure can overstimulate the mind, contributing to its busyness. Our meditation does not exist in a mental vacuum—the body is very closely related to it; everything that affects it affects our meditation. Do an honest self-appraisal and take care of your body's needs.

Practice

- - - - - - - - - -

TUNING YOUR PRACTICE

Think of your meditation as a guitar tuning process, where you are tightening and loosening the strings to find the right balance:

- When your mind is busy, switch for a time to an approach that best helps you slow and stabilize your mental activity—for example, increased concentration on an object of focus, longer exhales, lower body or chakra focus, body relaxing, calming affirmations, and so on.

- When your mind is drowsy, switch for a time to an approach that best helps you activate your mind in a guided way—such as inquisitiveness, longer inhales, upper body or chakra focus, body activating, movement, labeling.

- Whatever you choose, don't judge, self-shame, or overanalyze.

- When you are settled in a balance point, just let it be and let go.

Physical Pain or Illness

Many meditation traditions teach a specific meditation position, and some even consider an ability to sit in this position a prerequisite to learning to meditate. The most common is a cross-legged or "lotus" seated position with the hands resting on the knees or in the lap. Some traditions suggest sitting on the knees instead or involve mudras, sacred hand gestures that represent spiritual energies, qualities, or deities in Hindu traditions. These positions can cause physical discomfort until the body is used to them (and often even once it is!), and this pain can become a big distraction. If you have been meditating for a while, you may have found the perfect posture, but if you are experiencing discomfort, you may want to revisit your posture and focus on the most important factors. As we age, we often need to allow for changes in our body, something that many meditators may struggle with or overlook.

My advice if you are experiencing pain due to your meditation posture is simple: move. There is little value in sitting in continuous physical pain, and it can unnecessarily exacerbate arthritis and other joint issues. Forced rigidity can also be triggering for trauma survivors, something covered in chapter 3. However, some meditation traditions disagree and regularly counsel sitting through pain. The general argument for this is that by sitting with discomfort or perhaps examining or relaxing into it, we can discover that the true source of pain is our mind and learn to abide in equanimity even when it is present. This is certainly true, and I don't deny there can be value in working with discomfort, as well as with learning not to give in to every restless impulse our body produces. Above all, the value is really about finding balance so that meditation does not become harmful to your body, or a "macho" exercise in powering through.

To assess the balance for yourself, it's helpful to understand the roots of meditation positions. Physical yoga postures were originally designed as precursors to sitting meditation, designed to strengthen the body and align subtle energies within. We will talk more about the relationship between physical yoga and meditation in chapter 4, but it's important here to consider that the lotus position that has become the assumed meditation posture for many (or its more accessible cross-legged half lotus cousin) were originally normally taken after the body had already been warmed, stretched, and aligned through other postures. It wasn't necessarily a position a yogi would go into cold first thing in the morning.

As well, a meditation posture is much more than a physical position; it is representative of our mind state, and by aligning our body, our mind naturally settles into a calmer state. Will Johnson, in his book *The Posture of Meditation*, puts it this way:

> Ordinarily we think of meditation as an activity involving our minds, but in truth meditation is initiated by assuming a specific gesture with our bodies. This gesture or posture forms the literal base on which the focused inquiry of meditation ultimately rests and depends.[12]

Our meditation posture is a full-body gesture, or mudra; working toward aligning it is as important as working with our mind. Actually, working with our body *is* working with our mind. As seen previously, many strategies for dealing with busy or drowsy mind focused on the body.

If we discover tension or slouching in our body, we will discover it in our awareness as well; realigning our body will realign our mind. In this way, tuning our body—that is, refining our gesture—throughout our meditation may be as useful or even more so than working with our mind.

So what really matters in a meditation posture? While of course this varies amongst teachings, the common denominators are:

• **A solid, balanced base.** A cross-legged or lotus position creates a strong base from which you cannot easily topple. If you are in a chair, having your feet solidly on the ground is helpful. Either way, feeling balanced and solid on your sit bones is important.

• **An aligned spine.** This is ideal both physiologically and for aligning the energy body. Honor the natural curvature of your spine and let your head float gently atop it, without your chin jutting out or tucked rigidly

- - - - - - - - - - -

12. Will Johnson, *The Posture of Meditation: A Practical Manual for Meditators of All Positions*, (Boston: Shambhala Publications, 1996), 1.

in. Your shoulders should be open and relaxed—choose your hand positioning based on what best accomplishes this.

- **A relaxed but alert body.** Both of the above should be accomplished with the minimum amount of muscle tension necessary to do so. This may require the use of pillows behind your back or under your knees, which is fine; if possible, work toward gradually decreasing their use so that you can rest in this posture without them.

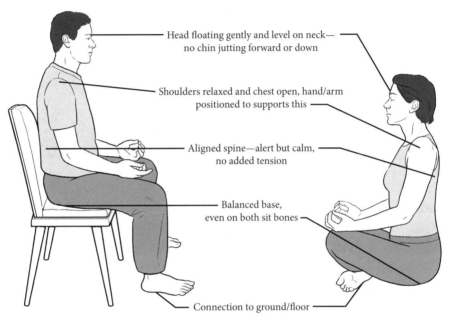

Head floating gently and level on neck—
no chin jutting forward or down

Shoulders relaxed and chest open, hand/arm
positioned to supports this

Aligned spine—alert but calm,
no added tension

Balanced base,
even on both sit bones

Connection to ground/floor

Figure 1: Meditation Body Alignment

Our meditation posture mirrors our mind state. If our mind is very busy or we are forcing our meditation in some way, our body will reflect this tension physically in the form of tight shoulders, a clenched or arched back, or jutted chin. If we are drowsy or spacey, our posture will usually collapse off balance to one side, our spine will slouch, or our chin will jut forward or down, breaking the alignment of our spine. Relaxing or re-aligning our body when we notice this triggers a corresponding shift in our mind state. Using this understanding of meditation posture as a guide, you can assess what aspects of your posture really matter, and work toward gradually improving them without regularly forcing yourself through pain. If you physically cannot sit in this way, let go of it. It can be an aid to your meditation but is *not* a requirement. Be understanding and compassionate with yourself!

As well, we may sometimes experience pain for other reasons, chronic or temporary, or become ill. While these may seem like major challenges to a meditation practice, they can also provide opportunities for exploring your relationship to discomfort. Working with pain and other symptoms through meditation in this way has been proven to be a valuable part of pain management programs, something we'll cover in more detail in chapter 3. Generally speaking, if you are working with pain either by choice in the case of working toward a more aligned meditation posture or due to injury or illness, consider trying one or more of the following:

- **Focus on the discomfort.** Our impulse is to move away or distract ourselves from pain or discomfort. Instead, allow your mind to rest on the pain itself. Become inquisitive. What is its size and shape? Does the feeling change as you focus on it? What is going on in your body around the pain?

- **Look into your feelings about the discomfort versus the discomfort itself.** Do you notice thoughts of "Will this ever stop?" or fear that it will worsen? Do you feel frustrated with the pain or illness? See if you can let these emotions go and just feel the pain.

- **Relax into the pain.** Experiment with this, and/or with relaxing one part of your body at a time. Notice any differences in your ability to relax when you get to the location in your body of the pain.

Working with meditation to help with chronic pain often requires professional support, but everyone can benefit from this kind of work to some extent. When we work with our discomfort, we are practicing nonreactivity. Our normal reaction is to do anything we can to remove the source of our discomfort, but this impulse does little for us when there is nothing we can change. To be in a body means sometimes experiencing pain or illness, and meditation can be a useful tool for learning how to accept it, relax into it, and extend ourselves compassion.

There are risks to working with pain in this way, however—it can trigger trauma reactions, or it can become a method for indulging in pain in a destructive or self-punishment pattern. A fellow yoga practitioner once described to me the way she had gone from self-harm through cutting as a teenager to what she called "extreme meditating" in her twenties where she forced herself to sit through pain in the name of practice. She was inspired by legends of yogis walking on hot coals without burning their feet and believed that meditating through pain would purify her through suffering. After a near breakdown, she entered therapy and realized how she had misused and misunderstood meditation. Fortunately, she received guidance in developing a balanced and healing new practice.

There are also risks associated with ignoring physical pain in meditation wherein it is used as a means to disassociate from the body entirely. Dissociation is covered in more depth later in the book; it can become an obstacle that twists a meditation practice into escapism and emotional bypassing rather than what it should do: lead us to greater presence and self-awareness. Feeling whole, present, and aligned in our body is our meditation ideal.

Practice

- - - - - - - - - - - -

WORKING WITH YOUR MEDITATION POSITION

- Assess your current meditation posture for the most important qualities (including pain). Determine if there are changes you would like to work toward.

- Experiment with focusing on your posture as a full-body mudra or gesture, tuning it instead of your mind as you meditate.

- If you are experiencing pain, illness, or discomfort that you cannot avoid, experiment with the various ways of reducing your resistance and changing your relationship to these sensations. Above all, be kind to yourself.

Life Happens

One of the biggest challenges to our practice can be changes in our routine, major life events, or serious life challenges. On some level, we know these are the times when we need our practice the most, but some part of us wants to put it off until conditions are better. We say, "I'll get back to my meditation when this deadline at work has passed/I'm done with this move/my mother is out of the hospital/the kids are back in school/I'm healed from my surgery/[fill in the blank]." Underlying this delay is a sense that our practice is part of an ideal life, some life other than the one we have now…that we'll get back to eventually. Of course, this isn't how life works, and often the best thing we can do for ourselves is let go of what our practice has looked like in the past and adapt it to what fits now.

I learned this lesson with the birth of my first child. I had children later in life; by the time my older daughter was born, I had been meditating an hour or more daily for sixteen years. My meditation time was sacred first thing every morning, and I even had a separate meditation room in which to practice. Of course, this all changed with a newborn baby who depended on me for her meals, was insistent upon her own schedule, and took over my formerly private space. In addition, six weeks after she was born, I suffered a severe gall bladder attack and had to undergo surgery, followed by two bouts of related infection, *and* the death of my stepmother. I craved my prior meditation routine and struggled with feelings of failure and resentment that I could not practice the way I had in the past. My meditation became a source of guilt, something I was never doing enough of, and consequently I could not settle into it when I was able to sit. Finally, an energy healer I was working with said to me, "Why are you meditating anyway? Why is there so much guilt? Right now, you need self-care, so cherish yourself in meditation, whether it's for five minutes a day or two hundred."

Her advice helped me shift the way I was relating to my meditation, and ultimately initiated me into a new more self-nurturing phase of practice. I let go of meditating in a dedicated place for a certain time for a set period. I practiced whenever or wherever I could: while nursing, waiting in a car for an appointment, or even in the shower. I focused on what I needed—energy, healing, or soothing—and shifted the form of my practice accordingly. I realized I'd been paying lip service to integrating my practice with daily life for years, and that in fact I had come to relate to it at times as a form of escapism and energetic empowerment. While eventually I was able to return to a more regular formal practice, this phase of practice—along with the tremendous opening of the heart that comes with parenthood—was life changing and helped me integrate my practice and life in ways I could never have anticipated.

While I am a big fan of a regular, formal, meditation routine and feel that with the demands of modern life most of us will not benefit from practice without regularity (a view borne out by research), I also think it's important to relate to your meditation as a form of self-care when you are struggling. Whenever you find yourself avoiding your meditation and saying "I'll get back to it when …," contemplate what you need now and practice *that* in your meditation. Stressed from a work deadline? Practice a relaxation method for five minutes a day. Healing from surgery? Do a healing light meditation when you can catch a few moments. Mourning the loss of a loved one? Practice self-compassion and maybe compassion for others also mourning. Find a meditation form that feels like medicine—a balm for your suffering. Don't worry if it doesn't look too formal. As co-founder of the Insight Meditation Society Sharon Salzberg says, "Meditation is the ultimate mobile device; you can use it anywhere, anytime, unobtrusively."[13]

Be aware that not all meditation traditions advise adapting your practice in this way, and there *is* value to committing to the same form of meditation and the same routine through any challenge or life event. Your practice becomes your ground, the one steady aspect of your life from which you can clearly see the transience of everything else, including the changes taking place within. You eventually let go of thinking in terms of enjoying or not enjoying your practice—it is just something you do, no matter what. I have certainly taken this approach too when life was in flux or I was facing challenges. It has shown me how our practice can be reborn over and over, within this one lifetime.

----

13. Sharon Salzberg, *Real Happiness: The Power of Meditation, a 28 Day Program,* (Workman Publishing Company, 2010), 21.

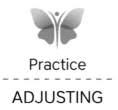

Practice

- - - - - - - - - - -

ADJUSTING

- Practice honest self-assessment. If life has thrown you a curve ball, see if you can find a way to turn *to* your practice, not away from it.

- If you can hold steady in your regular practice then great, but if not, ask yourself what you need from it right now, and embrace meditation as self-care. Allow it to adapt in form, place, and length.

- Do what you can do. Let your life and meditation inform each other, as they are meant to. Let go of guilt or "shoulds."

Contemplations

- What is your meditation routine, and are you satisfied with it? If you'd like to increase its regularity or length, which of the routine-building tips will you employ and how? What is your new goal?

- Have you tended to struggle more with drowsiness or busyness in your meditations? What methods do you use to work through each? Did you find any new methods listed here that you would like to try?

- If you consistently struggle with one of these more than the other, do you think it has roots in a larger emotional coping pattern that you need to explore and work with outside of meditation?

- Have you found a comfortable meditation posture for yourself that fulfills the main purposes of such a posture? If not, how might you change it based on those purposes? Do you feel the connection between your posture and your mind during your meditation?

- What has been your relationship to your meditation practice when major life events have occurred for you? Have you turned to it or away from it? How might you adapt your practice to the changing circumstances of your life?

THREE

THE SCIENCE OF MEDITATION

In the last thirty years it has sometimes seemed every week a new research study has been released extolling the benefits of meditation. This has been wonderful in that it has helped meditation go mainstream, and it is now taught in corporations, hospitals, schools, prisons, and more. However, it has also created unrealistic expectations that can sometimes be discouraging to practitioners when they don't immediately experience constant calm or perfect health. The results of a lot of past meditation studies are in fact now being reexamined as researchers realize they didn't always control for relevant external factors, fully describe the method of meditation individuals engaged in, account for the length of time participants had been meditating, and other factors. While I recognize the need for caution regarding claims about meditation in these reassessments, I find that reading about this research can help motivate and refine our practice. While in part II we will devote several chapters to exploring what *spiritual* traditions teach us about meditation, in this chapter we will cover a bit of what *science* has to teach us, including what it is able to measure—and what it is not.

Some of the most interesting recent research involves how meditation changes our brain. This is important because it confirms what spiritual traditions have long upheld—that meditation isn't just about relaxation or mystic experience but permanent positive personal change. As Daniel Goleman and Richard Davidson, two preeminent psychologists and researchers in this area put it, "It's not the highs along the way that matter. It's who you become."[14] Monitoring changes to our brain helps scientists understand not just *how* meditation benefits us, but *why*. As a meditator, understanding how you yourself are changing can help focus your practice.

One of the most compelling findings is that long term meditators have an increased amount of gray matter in parts of the brain linked to working memory, decision making, problem solving, and sensory processing.[15] The density of gray matter in any particular part of our brain maps to higher capability in the function that area of our brain is responsible for. Since the particular form these meditators had been practicing, insight meditation, involves focusing on sensory input and mental events, it's understandable that sensory capabilities would be enhanced. Of more surprise to researchers was the finding that the parts of the brain responsible for memory and executive functions like decision making and problem solving were denser, since these functions were not actually being used during meditation. In other words, this form of meditation didn't just strengthen the areas of the brain being utilized during practice, it also appears to have enhanced gray matter production in other important areas.

These findings were particularly interesting because normally our brain loses gray matter as we age, particularly in the area tied to memory and problem solving. But in this study, fifty-year-old long-term meditators had the same amount of gray matter in this brain region as twenty-five-year-old nonmeditators. In order to determine whether or not the long term meditators had simply started out with more gray matter, researchers conducted another study, this time comparing brain images of participants before and after an

- - - - - - - - - - - -

14. Daniel Goleman and Richard Davidson, *Altered Traits: Science Reveals How Meditation Changes Your Mind, Brain, and Body* (New York: Avery; Reprint edition, 2018), 40.

15. Sara Lazar, et al, "Meditation experience is associated with increased cortical thickness," *Neuroreport*, Nov 2005, 1893–1897. https://www.ncbi.nlm.nih.gov/pmc/articles /PMC1361002/.

eight week Mindfulness-Based Stress Reduction (MBSR) program compared to a control group.[16] Meditators were asked to meditate forty minutes a day during this time, although the average length of time was about half an hour.

In just eight weeks, the MBSR program participants' brains were thicker than the control group's in four areas:

- The left hippocampus, linked to learning, cognitive ability, memory, and emotional regulation associated with self-awareness. Thickening in this area is associated with improvement in all these functions.

- The posterior cingulate cortex, associated with our level of self-orientation and subjectivity, including our level of distraction from self-referential mental chatter. When this area of the brain is stronger, our mind is *less* likely to wander. We are better able to notice the thoughts or sensations arising for us without becoming identified with them.

- The pons area of the brain, located in the middle of our brain stem, where many neurotransmitters responsible for regulating brain activity reside. Thickening here is associated with improved sleep and physical functioning, among other things.

- The temporoparietal junction, linked to empathy, compassion, and placing our experiences in a larger frame of reference—perspective.

In addition to growth in these areas, the meditators experienced a *shrinking* in the area of the brain associated with anxiety and fear—the amygdala. This correlates to a reduction in stress levels, as when this area of the brain shrinks, we are less likely to respond by default to everyday situations as stressful.

While previous behavioral-based studies of meditation had already linked it to stress reduction, improved memory, better cognitive function, improved sleep, and many other benefits, the importance of this and similar recent studies is that it utilized brain imaging and was thus able to verify the actual brain changes correlated to these benefits. These imaging studies confirm that

- - - - - - - - - - -

16. Britta Holzel, et al, "Mindfulness practice leads to increases in regional brain gray matter density," *Psychiatry Research: Neuroimaging* 191, January 2011, 36-43, https: //www.sciencedirect.com/science/article/abs/pii/S092549271000288X?via%3Dihub.

meditation is not simply a product of consciousness or a source of experiences and insights—it is a tool for transforming our brain and even for slowing brain aging. In this sense it would appear certain forms of meditation are to our brain what exercise is to our body—if we do it properly and regularly, our brain will strengthen and stay healthy longer.

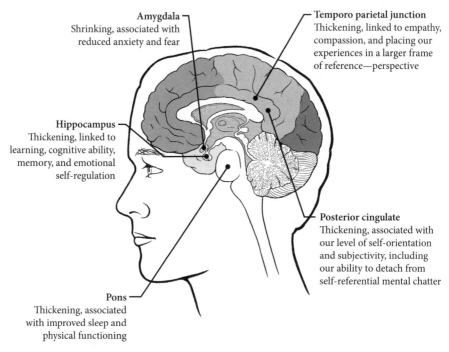

Amygdala
Shrinking, associated with reduced anxiety and fear

Temporo parietal junction
Thickening, linked to empathy, compassion, and placing our experiences in a larger frame of reference—perspective

Hippocampus
Thickening, linked to learning, cognitive ability, memory, and emotional self-regulation

Posterior cingulate
Thickening, associated with our level of self-orientation and subjectivity, including our ability to detach from self-referential mental chatter

Pons
Thickening, associated with improved sleep and physical functioning

Figure 2: Mindfulness-Linked Brain Changes

Mindfulness and insight forms of meditation have been the most re-searched in terms of these kinds of brain changes. This does not mean other forms do not yield these benefits, just that they have not yet been verified to do so. If you are interested in slowing the aging of your brain, thickening the areas of your brain associated with focus and present awareness, and/ or shrinking the areas associated with fear and anxiety, consider practicing these forms or adding them to your existing meditation routine. The mind-fulness practice included in chapter 1 is a great place to start, and the recom-mended book list has good resources for this too.

Changing Our Default

As I mentioned in the first chapter, meditation's stress management benefits stem not so much from inducing our body's relaxation response as from helping us shift our default relationship to thoughts, emotions, and even physical sensations. Depending on the form of meditation we practice, we either train in *noticing* these and letting them be, or we actively pull our mind away from them and back to our object of focus. Either way, we don't attach to whatever arises in our internal awareness stream, and this allows us to *choose* our response rather than simply react. Whether we experience anxiety, memories, or a pain in our knee, through meditation we train in nonidentification and in not reacting from identification.

Our default mode—reacting through identification—is linked to what neuroscientists call "self-referential mind-wandering," itself correlated to our brain's DMN (default-mode network). As we go about our day we spend most of our time in this mode, chattering to ourselves, identifying immediately with whatever is arising, and reacting. Research demonstrates that by meditating we can shift this default mode, reducing activity in our DMN, and shifting it to other areas of our brain associated with focus and present awareness. If we practice meditation enough, this shift continues outside of meditation, reducing our general level of mental chatter and reactivity.

In one study, researchers studied brain images before and after participants engaged in one of three different meditation forms—concentration, lovingkindness, and choiceless awareness. All three kinds of meditation reduced DMN activity and shifted brain activity to areas associated with greater self-regulation and cognitive control.[17] Furthermore, experienced meditators had lower baseline levels of DMN activity; their brains indicated that they were in self-referential mind-wandering mode less often than the control group, even when they weren't meditating.

This ability to shift our relationship to our thoughts and sensations is also at the heart of how meditation can help with pain management. It doesn't actually stop our physical pain, but it can help us change our relationship

- - - - - - - - - - - -

17. Judson Brewer, et al, "Meditation experience is associated with differences in default mode network activity and connectivity," PNAS 108, December 2011, 20254–20259, https://doi.org/10.1073/pnas.1112029108.

to our pain, and with time this can continue after meditation. Here's how a truck driver who was taught MBSR to help him deal with chronic pain describes this:

> No, the pain is not gone. It's still here, but you know when I start feeling it too much, I just sit aside somewhere, take ten, fifteen, twenty minutes, do my meditation, and that seems to take over. And if I can stay at least, say, 15 or 30 minutes or better, I can walk away and not even think about it for maybe three, four, five, six hours, maybe the whole day, depending on the weather.[18]

Similarly, meditation has been shown to help in addiction treatment, as participants are better able to "ride out" cravings when they arise. A specialized mindfulness program called Mindfulness-Based Relapse Prevention (MBRP) has been shown to be more effective than standard post-rehab support programs in helping prevent substance abusers who have undergone treatment from relapsing.[19] Similarly, a mindfulness program designed to help prevent relapses of depression was also shown to be more effective than standard programs. Participants were better able to withstand the kinds of triggering events and mood shifts that in other individuals might lead to a recurrence of depression.[20]

Programs designed to prevent relapse, in both the case of addiction and depression, coupled meditation with tools for changing and redirecting cravings or sadness. Participants were supported as they learned to *choose a different response* to these feelings. In other words, the first step was the non-reactivity developed through MBSR, and the second step was learning to choose a different response than in the past—a kind of self-reprogramming. This process is really at the heart of how meditation can fuel personal change of any

- - - - - - - - - - - -

18. Jon Kabat-Zinn and Richard J. Davidson, *The Mind's Own Physician: A Scientific Dialogue with the Dalai Lama on the Healing Power of Meditation,* (Oakland, CA: New Harbinger Publications, 2013), p. 41.

19. Anita Slomski, "Mindfulness-Based Intervention and Substance Abuse Relapse," *JAMA* 311, 2014; p. 7644. DOI:10.1001/jama.2014.7644.

20. Kabat-Zinn and Davidson, *The Mind's Own Physician,* 105.

type—learning to respond through conscious choice, *not* reactions from our old habits or ways of thinking. Whether we are working with pain, cravings, addiction, anxiety, anger, fear, unworthiness, shame, or any other emotional pattern, meditation can play a role in helping us to change our habitual mode as it is currently "written" into our brain. But to best do so, we need to focus on both aspects of change: strengthening our present awareness so we are not triggered into our old reactions, *and* cultivating replacement thoughts and activities, in an attempt to reprogram our old ways of being.

Mindfulness-based meditation practices are those most proven to help us with the former, and many other kinds of meditation can help with the latter including visualization, mantra, and affirmation-based forms, as well as chakra and energy meditations designed to cultivate positive emotional states. These are all examples of "practicing" a new state—actively cultivating it within a meditation through sound, symbol, vibration, or words. Balancing these two kinds of practice is often the best way to accomplish personal transformation, and when we focus on only one aspect or the other, we may not see the results we would like.

One example of this comes through the story of Amy, a social worker who had practiced MBSR daily for some time. She felt it had greatly improved her ability to choose caring emotional responses with both clients and friends. She felt less triggered and moody than before she meditated regularly. However, she was feeling stagnant and unable to manifest change in her life. She wanted to explore other career avenues and meet new people but felt stuck in the routine of her life and was having a hard time acting on these desires. She decided to try an online personal development course oriented around the law of attraction and personal change, something she had previously dismissed as flaky and wishful thinking. As part of this course, she was asked to meditate two different ways daily on the changes she wished to cultivate in her life: first, to imagine herself in a fulfilling new job and interacting with many new friends, and then to abstract from this the emotions and energy of that visual, and to imagine this energy filling her body to rest in this feeling for a time.

At first, Amy felt foolish engaging in this kind of work; it felt like simple daydreaming. But with time, the feeling of her visual began to seem more real to her, and she found herself more motivated and spontaneously thinking outside of meditation of ways she might reach her goals. She realized that during these sessions she actually was practicing feeling like a new version of herself, and it created momentum for her to move forward. She came to view her MBSR and this visualization practice as two complementary aspects of her personal transformation efforts. MBSR helped her recognize her current emotional patterns so that she was better able to disengage from them. Her visualization and affirmation work helped her imagine and eventually realize new emotional patterns, ones more in line with who she wanted to become and the life she wanted to have.

Personal development programs focused on variations of law of attraction teachings have become very prevalent and can be problematic—at times, they cross over into escapism or victim blaming, wherein individuals feel responsible for challenging life events or illnesses they cannot control. Some would dispute the idea that this kind of personal development work is meditation at all. In actuality, many traditional forms of meditation work with the mind in the same way. In the deity and mantra work found in some Buddhist and Hindu traditions, the goal is to experience oneself as possessing the traits and energies represented by those deities and mantras. In chakra and other energy-based meditations, the person cultivates positive emotions associated with open chakras. We are drawing upon our imagination in a similar way when we engage in compassion and lovingkindness meditations in which we visualize sending these energies out to others. In all of these cases, by first imagining feeling a certain way, we eventually come to feel that way for real. However, there can be issues with practicing these forms of meditation exclusively; I have certainly met individuals who became so caught up in imagining a positive future self that they were ignoring the dysfunction in their present. These imagination-based forms of practice can become a way of escaping rather than changing. Finding the right balance for yourself is key, and understanding the ways different meditation forms impact your mind and brain can help you to navigate this.

Practice

AFFIRMATION MEDITATION

As we've noted in this chapter, personal change is best supported when you take a two-pronged approach: (1) strengthen your ability to identify existing thought and emotional patterns tied to the behavior you'd like to change, and (2) cultivate new thoughts and responses. Mindfulness practices helps us with the first, while affirmation meditation is an example of the second. While changing patterns linked to addiction, depression, self-harm, or other serious mental health issues requires professional support, you can experiment with affirmation meditation for smaller changes:

- Develop an "I am" statement that represents the new thought or emotional response you would like to cultivate, make it situationally specific as possible, and phrase it in the affirmative, e.g., "I am calm and efficient when confronted with sudden work assignments," "I am centered and grounded when driving in traffic," "I am loving and wise when speaking with my teenager about something difficult."

- Repeat this phrase to yourself several times, and as you do so, imagine the associated feeling is spreading throughout your body. Really focus on cultivating the feeling, not only the thought.

- Sit in meditation on this feeling, settle into it, allow yourself to be overtaken by it. When your mind wanders, return to saying the phrase and feel into it again.

- If you like, visualize yourself in an actual relevant situation, feeling the way you now feel, and responding differently than you have in the past.

Trauma Sensitivity

Researchers have recently made great strides in understanding how trauma affects the brain; unsurprisingly, it is the opposite manner in which meditation affects it in many ways. Experiencing trauma tends to increase amygdala density, the part of our brain connected to feelings of fear and anxiety, whereas this same area becomes less active and dense through meditation. Trauma often also reduces capacity in our hippocampus and prefrontal cortex, connected with self-regulation, working memory, emotional response, and decision-making, and meditation has been shown to increase density in these areas.[21] Meditation would seem to be an excellent countering component of trauma treatment, and indeed it can be. But it is not a good fit for everyone, as some can find it triggering. If you have experienced trauma in your life or are introducing meditation to someone who has, it's very important to understand principles of trauma sensitivity in contemplative work.

Whether from abuse, an accident, assault, other violence, sudden illness, a natural disaster or profound loss, many of us experience some form of trauma in our lifetimes. If we include victims of secondary trauma (those affected by hearing about or witnessing the traumatic event of a family member, friend, patient, or client) and systemic trauma (living in a sustained stress-inducing environment including that fueled by poverty and/or bigotry) the numbers are even larger. Traumatic experiences overwhelm our system, creating breaks in our sense of reality that our psyche has difficulty integrating. When we aren't able to integrate, our trauma may manifest in any number of physical and emotional ways—we may become chronically anxious, unable to sleep, engage in dissociative behavior, experience flashbacks, or become triggered by seemingly mundane sounds and stimuli. Not everyone who experiences trauma will develop PTSD, but many will experience one or more of these issues at some point.

Meditation has become a valuable part of many trauma treatment programs, and some of the research into the brain described above explains why. However, there's a growing understanding that meditation can also become triggering, resulting in the exact opposite effect. Sometimes this happens immediately when a survivor learns to meditate, or sometimes meditation helps for a time but then problems begin to arise. As David Treleaven, author of *Trauma-Sensitive Mindfulness: Practices for Safe and Transformative Healing* explains:

---

21. Melanie Greenberg, "How PTSD and Trauma Affect Your Brain Functioning," *Psychology Today,* Sep 29 2018, https://www.psychologytoday.com/us/blog/the-mindful-self -express/201809/how-ptsd-and-trauma-affect-your-brain-functioning.

For people who have experienced trauma, mindfulness meditation can exacerbate symptoms of traumatic stress. This can
include flashbacks, heightened emotional arousal, and disassociation—meaning a disconnect between one's thoughts, emotions, and physical sensations. While meditation might appear
to be a safe and innocuous practice, it can thrust trauma survivors directly into the heart of wounds that require more than
mindful awareness to heal. By raking their attention over inju-
ries that are often internal and unseen, trauma survivors can
end up…disoriented, distressed, and humiliated for somehow
making things worse.[22]

The plethora of media sources telling us that meditation will help us feel
calmer and healthier actually contributes to this problem by making anyone
who doesn't experience this fearful they are failing or irreparably damaged.
Trauma survivors are often especially susceptible to these thoughts, leading
to increased feelings of isolation and hopelessness. But this kind of triggering can happen even if you don't consider yourself a trauma survivor. Meditation is often the only time we slow down; sometimes long-buried memories or feelings bubble up at these times for us to finally deal with. If this
happens to you, it is not a sign that something is wrong with you or that you
are meditating incorrectly—it is sometimes just the mind's way of showing
us what we need to focus upon in order to heal. It may also be a sign to slow
down, seek help, or shift our practice.

If you have experienced trauma in your life and/or find that troubling
emotions or memories are arising in meditation, try to find a professional
trained in trauma sensitivity to help you. (I have included several relevant
books, including Mr. Treleaven's quoted above, in the Recommended Book
List.) The handling of certain disturbances appears in chapter 7, but it's
important to recognize when you need support and seek it. If you do feel
able to experiment with your practice yourself, here are some basic suggestions for how you might do so:

- - - - - - - - - - -

22. David A. Treleaven, *Trauma-Sensitive Mindfulness: Practices for Safe and Transformative
Healing,* (New York: W.W. Norton and Company, 2018), 8.

- **Adapt.** If you find a traditional straight-backed posture, closed eyes, or focusing on the breath at all triggering, experiment with all of these. Instead of using the breath as an anchor for example, you might use the feeling of your feet on the floor as your meditation anchor or "object of focus," or even sounds or a visualization in your mind. Perhaps movement forms will be more comfortable for you. The important thing is to choose what works for you rather than feel constrained by a triggering form.

- **Focus on feelings of safety.** In terms of environment, length of time, whether to practice alone or in a group, or any other aspects of your meditation, select what feels safest to you personally, not based on what you think you "should" do. Perhaps dim lighting or incense, which others find relaxing, are actually uncomfortable for you—if so, don't use them or meditate in a setting in which they are present. Sit with your back to the wall if that feels better for you.

- **Self-nurture.** Also make feelings of safety primary in terms of which form of meditation you choose to practice. Select one that feels nurturing and healing. Do not feel as though you have failed if a particular form does not work well for you (and do not let anyone else make you feel this way). Honor your right to choose.

- **Wait on retreats.** More is not always better when it comes to meditation. Don't engage in a group or long retreat until you are sure you are ready, and let go of the idea you should "power through" any meditation. Allow yourself to honor what your body is telling you. Knowing when you are ready for retreat is covered in more depth in chapter 9.

- **Seek support.** Especially if you experience flashbacks as the result of meditation—either in a session or an increased amount in general once you have begun a meditation practice—seek qualified support. You may need to work with what is arising for you directly through another modality outside of meditation. We will talk more about integration and post-meditation practices later as they are a valuable part of any healing, personal growth, or spiritual journey.

As the spiritual traditions of the East and the psychological traditions of the West continue to intermingle and inform each other, more and more information is available as to how to adapt them both for the greatest benefit. Especially in the area of handling trauma, this is a very important development. If this is relevant to you, please be gentle and honor your healing process.

Practice

- - - - - - - - - - - -

TRAUMA CONSIDERATIONS

- If you have experienced trauma in your life and experience any form of triggering in your practice, don't try to push through it, or judge your meditation. Instead, work with the trauma sensitive principles above to adapt your practice and/or seek professional support.

- Even if you do not consider yourself a trauma survivor, recognize that at times meditation may facilitate the arising of difficult emotions or memories that your psyche has not had time to process before. Some of these are covered in chapter 7, but if you ever feel overwhelmed, seek support.

- Be kind and compassionate with yourself.

Compassion and Brain Changes

So far, most of the brain studies we have covered involved variations on mindfulness practice. But a series of University of Wisconsin studies related to compassion practice garnered big headlines for their finding that these practices also change the brain, essentially hardwiring it to be more compassionate overall.[23] The first studies involved measuring Tibetan monks' brain activity as they rotated between phases of compassion meditation and rest. Although these monks were experienced meditators, the researchers

- - - - - - - - - - -

23. Antoine Lutz, et al, "Regulation of the Neural Circuitry of Emotion by Compassion Meditation: Effects of Meditative Expertise," *PLOS ONE,* March 2008: 1897, https: //doi.org/10.1371/journal.pone.0001897.

expected it would take some time for them to enter into a focused, meditative state. Instead they saw a big burst of electrical activity right away at the start of each phase in which the monks were engaged in compassion meditation versus the rest periods. When examining brain scans, they confirmed that the areas of the brain associated with empathy did indeed light up—in some cases seven to eight hundred times higher than during the rest periods.

In addition, researchers discovered that the monks had highly elevated gamma brain wave emanations not only during meditation but during their everyday activities. One of the five brainwave states we shift between throughout our day—delta, theta, alpha, beta, and gamma—gamma is the fastest vibrating frequency and is associated with moments of great insight and creativity, characterized by the simultaneous and harmonious "firing" of regions throughout our brain. In most people, gamma wave bursts are infrequent and last only a second, not a normal state of being. In these monks, gamma levels had become the norm.

In a later study, the same researchers also taught a compassion practice to beginning meditators and compared their brain scans before and after. Although there are various compassion practice forms, in this one, participants were first asked to focus on sending thoughts of lovingkindness and wishes for well-being to family and friends, gradually expanding that out to more and more people, eventually sending it out to all beings unconditionally. After just two weeks, brain scans indicated activity in the same areas of the brain linked to compassion that had seen the most activity in the monks. The implications are clear: we can become more compassionate through this kind of meditation practice, it happens almost as soon as we begin practicing this form of meditation, and with time it can permanently change our brain's default and thus our way of being in the world.

Practice

- - - - - - - - - -

ENDING WITH COMPASSION

- You can incorporate compassion practice into your regular meditation by ending with sharing your practice. Simply imagine gathering up whatever peace, goodwill, or contentment you felt during your meditation and offer these moments outwards to all beings.

• Visualize this as a bundle of light that encapsulates your best moments. Focus on the feeling of magnifying and sharing these moments—you are not giving them away and *losing* them, you are sharing them with others as an act of compassion, and as you do so, imagine they become infinite and omnipresent in the world.

Check the Recommended Book List for resources on other forms of compassion practice.

Neuroplasticity and Epigenetics

The kind of brain changes covered here demonstrate neuroplasticity. Also known as brain plasticity, the term refers to the ability to forge new neural pathways and synapses in the brain due to changes in thinking, emotions, situations, and environment. For a long time, scientists believed our brains were relatively static after early childhood and real change at the neural level was not possible. We now know that profound changes can and do occur, and that they continue throughout our lifetime. Here are some examples of neuroplasticity:

• Stroke victims recovering lost functionality due to their brains reorganizing themselves so that new neural pathways take over functions previously performed by the damaged part.

• Deep sea divers seeing hundreds of feet deep underwater because they have learned to control their eye lenses and pupils through brain control the rest of us never develop.

• Professional musicians' brains developing extra gray matter in the areas of the brain related to playing their instruments—so much so that neuroscientists can often identify a professional musician by looking at a scan of their brain.

• Athletes' visualizing perfect performance, and brain scans showing this strengthens the same parts of the brain that are activated when they are actually physically performing.

• All of the examples from the prior sections of this chapter involve neuroplasticity—meditators' brains developing *more* gray matter in areas associated with self-regulation, memory, cognitive function, and compassion, and *less* gray matter in areas associated with anxiety and fear, as well as increased gamma ray activity in experienced meditators' brains when engaged in everyday activities (which involves harmonious neural activity throughout the entire brain).

These examples all serve as proof that the brain changes in response to our environment, activity, or thoughts. Our thoughts change our brain; our brain doesn't simply determine our thoughts. While this may sound pretty fundamental to anyone involved in mind-body modalities, it was a revolution in neuroscience. And of course, it means you can change your brain—and thus your body—through the power of your mind, including through meditation.

We've already outlined the ways mainstream science has sought to measure these changes. But there are a lot of meditation modalities whose impact aren't as easily measurable—at least not yet, in a way that is widely acknowledged by academia. Energy-based forms such as kundalini meditation, chakra focus, subtle body visualizations, and release techniques approach thoughts and emotions as energy, or vibration, and involve working directly at this level. As our vibration changes and opens channels within our subtle body, these traditions assert we are changed at our cellular level to include physical healing as well as the release of negative emotional and mental patterns that are replaced with healthier, happier ones. Our subtle body is considered a link between mind and body—we visualize or focus on a particular chakra or location in our subtle body with our *mind* and feel it in our *body*.

It is not only explicit energy-based traditions of meditation that acknowledge this vibratory aspect of meditation; it is part of mindfulness and insight traditions as well. As Jack Kornfield, one of the key Western Buddhist teachers to introduce mindfulness in the West, put it at a conference between researchers and the Dalai Lama:

> "…there is an intensive meditative training that shows us how to experience the world as vibrations. When attention

to this level becomes highly developed and the mind concentrated, sound is experienced as a series of vibrations at
the ear and then at the heart. Then sight and thought can
be experienced as vibrations. You can even sense yourself
about to think…It would be interesting to study subjects
who've learned how to deliberately synchronize their inner
vibrations or in some way work with the vibratory aspect of
consciousness."[24]

Future chapters will cover this level of meditation in more depth, but
within the context of this chapter it's interesting to surmise what working
at these subtle levels of mind and body might mean in terms of healing and
personal growth. If we can change our brain through meditating, could we
change our genes, for example? The burgeoning field of epigenetics says we
just might be able to. Epigenetics is the study of what factors affect how a
given gene in our DNA sequence expresses itself. For example, we may have
a genetic propensity for a particular medical problem but never manifest that
problem. Which lifestyle, diet, and environmental factors affect whether that
genetic tendency does or doesn't manifest? This, in a nutshell, is the study of
epigenetics. The particular aspects of our DNA that do manifest during our
lifetime is more fluid than we ever thought.

One of the more groundbreaking findings within epigenetics is that some
changes may actually be passed down between generations. There is already
research to suggest that trauma in particular alters gene expression and makes
us more prone to health problems later in life. Now there is also research that
suggests this gene expression may in fact be handed down to future generations, i.e. trauma in one generation negatively affects the health of future generations. On the plus side, there is the possibility that healing from trauma,
reversing the gene expression and manifesting good health and psychological
effects will also flow down to the next generation. In other words, when we
heal, we heal not only ourselves but *future generations* too.

Mainstream science is a long way from connecting the findings of neuroplasticity and epigenetics, and for the most part it does not acknowledge

- - - - - - - - - - -
24. Kabat-Zinn and Davidson, *The Mind's Own Physician*, 126.

the power of energy healing and techniques to manifest physical change. But looking at current meditation research, it's hard not to get a sense that science is on the brink of validating what many spiritual and energy healing traditions have taught for centuries: that we have the power to change and heal at any point in our lives, that how we choose to live and the states of mind (or vibration) that we choose to manifest impacts our body, brain, and even genes, and that this carries forward beyond ourselves to future generations and thus the future of our world.

Practice
ENERGY AWARENESS

- Explore the way your energy or vibratory level shifts during your meditation by checking in at the beginning and end of your formal practice. If this is new for you, begin by simply tuning in briefly to your body and choose one word that best describes your overall state: tense, tired, irritable, relaxed, alert, et cetera.

- Now describe for yourself the nature of this state as an abstract energy— is it dense or wispy, placid or frenetic, big or small, static or moving, warm or cold, clear or opaque? While this may at first seem unfamiliar, with time you will develop your energetic sensitivity through this method.

- Do this again at the end of your meditation, and see if new words arise, and how you would describe them energetically. Eventually you can jump directly to the energetic description.

Checking in before and after your meditation through this method can help you to discern the subtler ways your practice affects your vibratory state. Often, we focus on how focused we felt or what we did or didn't think about and subsequently miss these subtle shifts.

What Science Can't Measure (Yet!)

For all the progress science has made, it cannot yet fully explain the most fundamental aspect of being human—consciousness. We can measure how different experiences in our consciousness reflect in our brain, but we cannot explain our ability to be conscious of them in the first place. We therefore cannot explain—or explain away—the mystic experiences we might have in meditation, although scientists have identified the parts of the brain activated during them. Dr. Andrew Newberg, a leading researcher in the field of neurotheology, which studies the relationship between the brain and religious experience, puts it this way:

> We can't tell you the origin of the [mystic] experience. But we can tell you the brain does appear to be built to have these experiences. There are examples of people reaching similar states, spontaneously. But for the most part, it takes work. Meditation and these powerful prayer experiences require dedication and practice. But people have figured out how to do this, and the question is, "What is the source of that experience?" The answer is, "We don't know." Science doesn't really have an answer for you.[25]

In his research, Newberg and his partner reviewed brain scans of both Tibetan monks in meditation and Franciscan nuns in prayer and compared the images at the peak of their practice. In both cases, the activity in the brain responsible for orienting ourselves in space as separate from the objects around us—an area of the brain normally always "on"—was greatly diminished. The feelings of oneness and boundarylessness described by both the monks and nuns were reflected in their brain as diminished activity linked to self-orientation and separation from surroundings. However, although both groups described their experience in fairly similar terms and their brains scans showed similar results, the two groups interpreted their experiences very differently. While the Tibetan Buddhist monks described it as a

----

25. Steve Volk, *Fringe-ology: How I Tried to Explain Away the Unexplainable—And Couldn't*, (New York: HarperOne, 2011), 181.

oneness or interdependence with all existence, the nuns described it as a feeling of closeness and intimacy with God. Both groups integrated their experience within the context of their specific religious backgrounds.[26]

As Newberg points out, science has a long history of pathologizing religious experience; for example, some posit that historic saints' mystic moments were the results of epilepsy or mental illness. His studies at the very least demonstrate that our brain naturally possess the capacity for spiritual experience, and the fact that we then interpret those experiences within varying philosophical or theological frameworks does not invalidate them.

Newberg also studied how spiritual experience reflected within participants' nervous systems and limbic system (linked to our emotions). From this perspective, he identifies four categories of spiritual experience:

- Hyperquiesence—deep relaxation and tranquility, related to the parasympathetic nervous system
- Hyperarousal—powerful alertness and concentration, a feeling of being in a "flow," related to the sympathetic nervous system
- Hyperquiesence with Arousal Breakthrough—deep absorption leading to bliss; within it the sympathetic and parasympathetic nervous systems are both activated, which is normally not the case
- Hyperarousal with Quiescent Breakthrough—ecstatic waves of energy leading to deep stillness; also characterized by interactions between sympathetic and parasympathetic nervous systems

These states are achievable through both active and passive forms of spiritual practice. He characterizes active forms as concentration and object-based, where we initially orient around focusing on an object of meditation, e.g., our breath, a chakra, a deity, a mantra, or a prayer. Passive forms involve clearing the mind by releasing any identification with thoughts or stimuli as they arise in our consciousness—objectless meditation. One of the interesting aspects of his work is how closely the various neurological states he identifies map to classic texts' descriptions of meditative stages, termed the

----

26. Andrew Newberg and Eugene D'Aquili, *Why God Won't Go Away: Brain Science and the Biology of Belief,* (New York: Ballantine Books, 2001), 98–127.

samadhis within Hindusim and the *jnanas* in Buddhism. (We will cover these stages in the next two chapters.)

Before we move from science to these spiritual explanations of meditation, let's take a moment to review what science can tell us. Meditation changes our brain and by extension our default mode of being in the world. It really is practice…for greater self-awareness, compassion, mystic union, or all of the above depending on the forms we engage in. It may not always feel that way, such as when we pull our mind back for the tenth time from our to-do list or biggest problems—but it is. Valuing and trusting in this longer-term shift, regardless of the day to day experience, is perhaps the most important gift we can give ourselves when it comes to meditation.

Contemplations

- What brain changes is the form of meditation you practice linked to? Have you noticed any changes in your default behavior that might be attributed to your meditation?

- Did reading about the scientific research on meditation trigger you to want to try another form or adapt your own? How might you adapt your practice to better facilitate positive changes?

- What benefits did you read about that were new to you, if any?

- What are your current beliefs regarding that which science cannot yet explain—the source of human consciousness and the content of mystic and spiritual experiences?

PART II
MEDITATION FOR
THE SPIRITUAL SEEKER

In the course of history, meditation developed within spiritual traditions. As such, the most comprehensive information about what we might experience and how we might progress is found within them. It's common for many Westerners to initially meet meditation in a secular setting—a mindfulness or yoga class. But mindfulness practices stem from Buddhism, and yogic forms of meditation from the Vedas, the most ancient texts of Hinduism. While many world religions incorporate contemplative practices, these two traditions have the richest and most robust teachings, and so we will spend chapters 4 and 5 exploring some of these. In chapter 6 we'll briefly explore how mystics within other religious traditions have conceptualized the meditation journey, including within kundalini yoga, ancient Egyptian mysticism, Kabbalah, Catholicism, and Sufism.

Each of these traditions offer us a map of the spiritual maturation or realization process as it unfolds through meditation. There are stages we progress through and specific experiences we might have. While it's important to respect the differences between traditions and not conflate them, there are a lot of common elements, especially in terms of the role meditation plays. In general, within all of them:

- Spiritual progression involves shifting from our usual material level of consciousness to a subtler/lighter level. Although intellectual study may prepare us for these shifts, the subtler states aren't knowable through our intellect—we must experience them through meditation/contemplation.

- Intellectual and self-study *are* necessary, though, as complements to meditation to assure we integrate our experiences correctly.

- Meditation experiences are not the end goal, but part of the process—both preparatory and purifying on the way to spiritual realization.

- At some point we must "descend" or face our subconscious or shadow side—that is, honestly acknowledge our more disturbing traits and patterns, as these are the root of our greatest obstructions to spiritual growth.

- Our ethical behavior and actions within the world are just as important as our meditation practice, and in fact our lives on and off our cushion are entwined.

Even if your motivation for meditating is not spiritual, learning about some of the states of awareness described in traditional texts may be very helpful to you and possibly even open you to new ways of thinking about your meditation. If you already meditate within a particular tradition, hearing about others' maps may place your experiences in a new context. I have met many individuals who read about a particular meditation stage as described in a spiritual text and realized they had already had that experience but didn't have a way of processing it at the time. Some people experienced these states spontaneously as children, or as adults outside of meditation, and having a framework for understanding them now is helpful.

Of course, entire books (and series of books!) have been written about each of these traditions, so this section isn't meant to be a comprehensive guide to them. As always, the Recommended Book List contains resources for you to explore further. My focus here is to highlight the principles and wisdom that may be relevant to any meditator. The Practices and Contemplations include ways this material can be useful to you.

FOUR

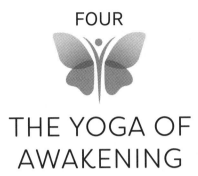

THE YOGA OF AWAKENING

It feels like I am part of everyone and everything in existence.[27]

I was no longer in my previous customary state but was led to find a peace in which I was united with God and was content with everything.[28]

I experience deep, unbounded silence, during which I am completely aware and awake, but no thoughts are present ... I feel completely whole and at peace.[29]

Three contemporary spiritual practitioners uttered these descriptions of their meditations—a Tibetan Buddhist, a Franciscan nun, and a serious student of a yogic meditation path—but their words could just as easily have come from a mystic in another century, or another tradition. Mystics throughout history have described their experiences in terms of wholeness, peace, and above all, union. It is the path to these experiences that yoga

---

27. Andrew Newberg and Eugene D'Aquili, *Why God Won't Go Away: Brain Science and the Biology of Belief,* (Ballantine 2001), 2.

28. Ibid., 7.

29. Frederick Travis and Craig Pearson, "Pure Consciousness: Distinct Phenomenological and Physiological Correlates of Consciousness Itself," *International Journal of Neuroscience* 100, March 1999: 77–89, https://doi.org/10.3109/00207450008999678.

teachings are meant to lay out for us, and in fact the word *yoga* means "yoke" or "union." In this chapter we'll explore the eight limbs of yoga as described by Patanjali in his *Yoga Sutras,* the foundation for classical yoga and the most well-known and translated yogic text. Although yoga's roots are in ancient India, many of the writings on meditation found within yogic teachings have relevance to any meditator. Patanjali was the first in a long line of yogis to lay out the meditative journey in a structured, almost scientific way that is more focused on practice than theology.

First the background: Patanjali lived somewhere between the second and fourth century CE, several hundred years after the Buddha, and many historians consider the *Yoga Sutras* to be heavily influenced by Buddhist monastic teachings. However, yoga overall predates Buddhism—Buddha was born in India and practiced meditation under yogic masters prior to the enlightenment that led to his teaching. Although there is debate about who Patanjali actually was and whether the *Yoga Sutras* was even written by just one person, we'll forgo that debate and work with the material in terms of its relevance to your practice.

Patanjali's eight limbs of yoga, which comprise just one part of the *Yoga Sutras,* are the path to spiritual union. Union with what? God, source, light, the absolute, ultimate reality, cosmic consciousness—various translations have all used these words. Another common one is Self with a capital "S," as opposed to lower case "self"; this model captures the essence of the yogic purpose, to merge (unite) our individual sense of self, our "I," into the infinite Self of all that is. This merging enables *moksha,* or liberation, as it is egoic delusions and hindrances that prevent us from knowing our self as Self in the first place. As we release these delusions and hindrances through our yoga practice, we are freed—enlightened.

The eight limbs of yoga are a path to this liberation, and what most of us would consider to be meditation comprises just three of the eight limbs. These limbs are presented sequentially, often as steps on a ladder, but I prefer to show them as a circle because together they form an integrated path—that is, we still practice the first limbs when practicing the eighth. As well, the circle shows how the limbs start externally and gradually move us inward. We begin by governing our outer behavior through self-restraint and gradually move inward, towards our true essence, as we engage in meditation and come closer to spiritual union. Although we focus on an "object" as part of our meditation practice, and this object becomes our conduit for experiencing union, the union is never really with something outside ourselves. In this sense, enlightenment is not actually a union at all but a discovery of our innermost core that has been there all along. Some metaphors used to describe this include a molecule of water dropped into the ocean, or a bottle breaking and the air once inside becoming indistinguishable from the air outside. Our true essence is already inside, and we work through the eight limbs of yoga, from the outermost in, to realize this.

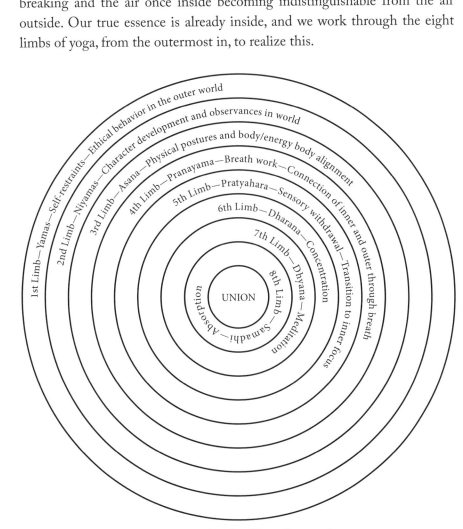

Figure 3: Eight Limbs of Yoga, Outer to Inner

Limbs one through four are sometimes referred to as preparatory for meditation—ethical living, character development, physical yoga, and breathing techniques. These each gradually draw us inward, culminating in the transition limb that is the fifth—sense withdrawal, consciously shifting our focus from the world "out there" to our internal landscape. In the sixth limb we begin concentration practice, which develops into true meditation, the seventh limb. Through proper practice we reach the eighth limb—the samadhis, or meditative absorptions.

However, even the samadhis are not liberation. If we improperly relate to the experiences of samadhi, if we attach to them, or upon leaving them lapse in the practice of any of the other seven limbs of yoga, we will not achieve union. Only through surrendering our attachments to these states and our sense of "I" entirely do we merge, shifting our identification from self to Self. Once this occurs our path is not about what we experience in meditation—it is our way of being.

In this way, the yogic path as Patanjali lays it out is both progressive and integrated. We can't practice one limb without the others, and meditation is just one piece. Enlightenment is also presented as both our natural state and hard work—there is nothing to attain, and yet there are stages to getting there. Being able to hold this paradox lightly is another key to walking the path with integrity.

First and Second Limbs—Ethics and Character

The first limb of yoga according to Patanjali is *yama*, usually translated as morality or self-restraint. Yama is ethical behavior in relation to others, and its five elements are non-violence in thought, word and deed (*ahimsa*), truthfulness (*satya*), non-stealing (*asteya*), celibacy or ethical use of our energy (*brahmacharya*), and non-greed (*aparigraha*). There are, of course, many commentaries on what these entail in daily life, but the essence could be considered to act considerately, not solely from self-interest in our relationships with others and the world. Can we tell the truth when it does not benefit us, avoid hurtful words or actions even when triggered, not misuse our sexual energy, steal, or accumulate just for the sake of satisfying our own desires?

These moral codes are similar to those of many other spiritual traditions but take on a different significance within the context of a yogic path. While the measure of our morality is based on external behavior, the real point is actually our internal relationships with others. Forcing ourselves to behave a certain way even though we feel otherwise is not really the point. If, as we traverse the path, we truly come to experience ourselves as merged and in union with all that is, then it would include others. After all, why would we then hurt, deceive, or covet? Working on our internal attitude toward others is the actual goal. As Patanjali puts it elsewhere in the sutras, "Undisturbed calmness of mind is attained by cultivating friendliness toward the happy, compassion for the unhappy, delight in the virtuous, and indifference towards the wicked."[30]

This is also true for the second limb, the *niyamas*, which involve character development, study, and the observance of spiritual rituals. The five elements of niyama are: cleanliness (*saucha*), contentment (*santosha*), discipline and enthusiasm (*tapas*), self and spiritual text study (*svadhyaya*), and contemplation of ultimate reality or a higher power (*isvara pranidhama*). Many yogic teachings contain specific cleansing or spiritual rituals related to cultivating the niyamas, but the real essence is turning the mind inward and cultivating a mindset conducive to spiritual growth. Cleanliness is not only keeping our home orderly and clean (though it does include this), it's about an orderly, clean state of awareness. Contentment arises when we cultivate non-attachment and presence and stop grasping at future goals or accumulations as the source of happiness. Discipline and enthusiasm are also extensions of this as inner attitudes brought to every task. Studying ourselves and studying spiritual texts prepares our mind to comprehend and integrate meditative experiences when we begin to have them, as does contemplation of the ultimate reality. Although this study is intellectual rather than experiential, it prepares us to properly understand what's to come, and once we begin to experience Self or consciousness—the ultimate reality—in meditation, it aids us in processing it correctly.

As we observe yama and niyama, they become automatic, no longer requiring effort. Over time this leads to changes in the actual karmic levels of our mind—what we experience as instinct. What once required effort

--- --- --- --- --- --- --- --- --- ---

30. Swami Prabhavananda and Christopher Isherwood, *How to Know God: The Yoga Aphorisms of Patanjali*, (Vedanta Press, 1950), 66.

is now innate. Swami Satchidananda, another prominent Indian yogi who brought yoga to the West, explains this process of change this way:

> Yoga says instinct is a trace of an old experience that has been repeated many times and the impressions have sunk down to the bottom of the mental lake. Although they go down, they aren't completely erased…when the proper atmosphere is created, they come to the surface again. When we do something several times it forms a habit. Continue with that habit for a long time, and it becomes your character. Continue with that character and eventually, perhaps in another life, it comes up as instinct.[31]

This teaching points to a deeper purpose of yama and niyama—the purification of our karmic levels of mind. Every thought, word, and action leave an imprint on us that affects our overall state of awareness as well as the state of awareness brought to meditation. If we consider it our starting point, these outer practices contribute to our ability to meditate by helping us clear patterns that might hinder us in practice.

This principle is not an abstract one; it's easy to see that if someone is rude to you and inwardly you cannot maintain equanimity, you will become angry. That anger has a momentum that might continue for some time, most likely in the form of angry thoughts in your mind, perhaps also tension in your emotions and body. If you were previously in a good mood, it's now gone. If you sit down to meditate in this state, you may spend much of your meditation attempting to let go of these feelings and thoughts. Your state is *karma*, in the short term. In the long term, the more time you spend in angry states of mind, the more likely you are to become angry again, a tendency (in this case, to become angry) that forms *samskara*, or habit of mind. To put it in Satchinananda's terms, anger is now instinct and part of your character.

If instead you were able to inwardly stay calm in the face of this rudeness, you can let the event go. This doesn't mean you just put up with it—you can respond firmly from a calm place, and sometimes this is appropriate. But

--- --- --- --- --- --- ---

31. Swami Satchinananda, *The Yoga Sutras of Patanjali: Commentary on the Raja Yoga Sutras*, (Buckingham, VA: Integral Yoga Press, 2012), 92.

then what's done is done. The event is over for you, and you don't carry it with you. It does not impact your mood, it does not sink into your psyche, and your instinct and character are not shifted towards anger. When you sit down to meditate, you are free and clear. This is the link between inner attitude, samskaras, and karma, and between karma and our meditation. Yes, meditation can help us to work out negative emotions, and sometimes that's what a session is—we are working through anger or some other difficulty. But through ethical behavior, and striving to cultivate the inner qualities that make this ethical behavior automatic, we also purify our karma—we release obstructive samskaras and prevent the development of more—and this allows us to bring a calmer, quieter, more focused state of awareness into our meditation.

Practice

- - - - - - - - - - -

YAMA AND NIYAMA

- Select one yama or niyama to focus on for one week. I find two of the most accessible for this purpose to be the yama of non-lying or the niyama of cleanliness.

- Selecting just one will allow you to really observe how focusing intently on this external practice in your life affects your internal state. They are both harder than you might think, and part of the value of working with them is contemplating what does and does not constitute fulfillment of them. For example, is telling a white lie to spare someone's feelings or ignoring dust bunnies under your dresser okay?

- The examples listed here are mundane, but the main takeaway is to notice how focusing on your yama/niyama affects your overall mind state. If you like, journal daily about how things are going.

Third and Fourth Limbs—Postures and Breathing

Considering how extensive the practice of physical yoga (*asanas*), the third limb, has become in our contemporary world, Patanjali devotes amazingly few words to it. Our asana should be "seated in a position which is firm but relaxed." He offers a little more advice for attaining this, in terms of "relaxing or loosening effort and allowing attention to merge with the infinite."[32] Although Patanjali does not include specific physical postures or instruction on asana other than this, we know the following: yoga postures were practiced by yogis prior to and during his time, most were handed down teacher to student and expanded upon in each new generation, and these teachings evolved into the many yoga styles we know today. Asanas are a wonderful form of exercise, but that is not their only purpose; as best expressed by twentieth-century yogi B.K.S. Iyengar: "It is through the alignment of the body that I discovered the alignment of my mind, self, and intelligence."[33]

We've covered the importance of posture already in chapter 2, and the essential point is that mind and body are not separate. Cleansing and aligning one aids the cleansing and aligning of the other. In physical yoga we do more than stretch and tone—we purify and practice all of the yamas and niyamas as well. The attitude we bring to our postures and our fellow yogis is our inner practice. On a subtler level too, asanas developed not only to help us strengthen and detoxify our physical body *and* subtle body, the chakras and channels (*nadis*) that compose our energy anatomy. As the intersection between mind, body, and spirit the deepest levels of our subtle body are the repository for our samskaras—those impressions left by our thoughts, words, and deeds that compose our karma—and proper asana practice aids our release of these impressions.

The fourth limb, pranayama or breath practice, is accordingly often taught together with asana. *Prana* means "life force," an accurate description of breath and breathing as the body's foundational cycle. When we are stressed our breath quickens, when we are calm it slows—our breathing patterns reflect our mental and emotional state. The reverse is also true: we can work with our breath to affect our mind. Some pranayama techniques calm the mind, others energize it, and still others purify. The mastery of breathing techniques is entwined with asana practice as preparation for meditation or even for use

- - - - - - - - - - - -

32. Swami Prabhavananda and Christopher Isherwood, *How to Know God: The Yoga Aphorisms of Patanjali*, (Los Angeles: Vedanta Press, 1950), 150.

33. B.K.S. Iyengar, *Light on the Yoga Sutras of Patanjali*, (London: Thorsons, 1994), 22.

during it—simple pranayama techniques that related to working with a busy or drowsy mind appeared in chapter 2.

Focusing on our breath during physical yoga also strengthens the link between mind and body—we relax muscles with our exhale and extend further with our inhales. Through this interplay we discover our inner and outer balance points. Physical balance postures demonstrate this—try standing on one leg when your mind is aggravated or when you are holding your breath and you will quickly discover the connection. Calmness and ease of mind and breath are linked to physical balance, and it is through practicing external physical balance that we discover inner mental balance. As contemporary yoga teacher Shiva Rea describes it: "Balancing in yoga and life is a reflection of our inner state. Can we dance with change? Can we fall and try again with playfulness? Do we have the focus, skill, and attunement to find the still point within it all?"[34]

Whether or not you practice asana or pranayama, you can work with your body and breath in this way. Many mind-body modalities such as tai chi, qi gong, martial arts, Pilates, and even dance employ the link between mind, body, and breath. You can bring it into any exercise form to some extent. Exploring this interrelationship, and what it means to find the "still point" Shiva Rea describes, can only help your meditation practice, and help you to integrate what arises there into your life.

Practice

BEGIN WITH THE BODY

- If you have a yoga practice and do not normally meditate afterwards, experiment with doing so. See if you can feel the difference in your awareness state.

- If this is not possible, try doing one or two basic poses at the very least before your meditation, and work with your breath as well. See if you

34. Shiva Rea (@shivarea108), Instagram photo and quote, April 30, 2011, https://www .instagram.com/p/pHA_8YPInH/?igshid=1naqbcshy7z8b.

can notice how working with your body and breath in this way begins to shift your awareness and prepare you for meditation, serving as a transition state.

- If you do not have a yoga practice, you can still experiment. Before your meditation, stand with your feet planted hip-distance apart. Take a deep, cleansing breath inward while raising your arms. Then exhale while slowly lowering your arms. Do this five to ten times, then sit down to meditate.

- Do you notice a difference? Experiment with the deep breathing over a couple of days and you will likely begin to discover the connection between physical movement, breath, and mental settling. To some extent you can use almost any form of exercise or movement in this way (though mind-body modalities such as yoga are specifically developed for it).

Fifth and Sixth Limbs—Drawing Inward and Concentration

With the fifth and sixth limbs we finally begin to practice what we might consider to be meditation, although within Patanjali's system it's only meditation if we reach the next limb, full concentration or *dhyana*. In his system, the fifth and sixth limbs, *pratyahara* (sense withdrawal) and *dharana* (concentration), are still considered preparatory steps, but the practices included within them would today conventionally be considered forms of meditation. Pratyahara is often described as turning the mind and *prana* inward, countering its default tendency to reach outward in engagement with the world. In our contemporary culture, this turning inward can be especially challenging, as our senses are constantly bombarded; the daily pace for most of us is not conducive to turning away from it. But turning away is the first step in meditating, one we repeat—that pulling of the mind away from everything it encounters and our own discursive thought.

Pratyahara is often understood to require physical separation from sensory input, and of course it is important to take breaks from stimuli and create a dedicated meditation spot that limits our distractions when developing a meditation practice. Pratyahara is also about our internal relationship to stimuli, and in some ways pratyahara can be compared to mindfulness. We turn inward to *notice* what is going on, which then helps us develop nonreactivity. This activity is not exclusive to physical stimuli or the sights and sounds around us as we meditate—it also includes our relationship with our own thoughts, which are themselves often reaching outward—the imaginary conversations with people in our lives, fantasies or longing for a future moment, or focus on something we do or don't want (a hope or fear). Through pratyahara, we inwardly pull away from all this activity, external and internal, and create some space. Within this space we can practice nonreactivity, and of course in this sense pratyahara is not only something we practice in sitting meditation. As with the first four limbs, practicing it throughout our daily lives carries over into our meditation and vice versa.

The sixth limb, dharana or concentration, follows naturally from the pulling inward of the previous limb. We of course practice concentration in the prior limbs too, especially in asana (postures) or pranayama (breath work). But when doing physical yoga or breath exercises, our mind is shifting from one focus to another, e.g., making body adjustments or counting the seconds of our inhales and exhales. With dharana we shift to *single-pointed* attention with a consistent meditative object of focus. The object itself is not very important here; for our purposes, it could be a mental image of a deity, a candle flame, a mantra, a chakra, or the breath. In later limbs, the difference in this object of focus *does* matter—what we focus on may determine which initial samadhis we experience. But at the level of the sixth limb, what matters is that focusing helps us develop concentration. Patanjali sees concentration as practice fixing or holding our mind onto *one* thought, a singular thought of our object. We grab hold mentally to our object of focus; as we stop the usual constant movement of the mind, the object serves as an anchor.

As we experience longer periods of our mind anchored in this way, we may slip into periods of true meditation, or as Patanjali defines it, the seventh limb of *dhyana*. We will talk more about this in the next section, but it's important to understand that this happens naturally each time our mind settles, and that we may go in and out of dhyana. These periods of dhyana are when we are most likely to begin to experience the pleasurable states sometimes associated with meditation—calmness, peace, contentment, or joy.

Although the drawing inward of the fifth limb and the concentration of the sixth are presented as preparatory to the seventh limb of true meditation, in actuality we are working with all three of these levels and possibly the eighth, samadhi, every time we sit down to meditate. We don't simply master a level one day and start where we left off the next time we sit down. One day we may spend our entire meditation stabilizing the fifth and sixth limbs, pulling our mind back to our object of focus over and over. Another day, more likely if we've been practicing awhile, we may begin to have days where we stabilize enough at these levels to experience brief periods of true dhyana/meditation or even a samadhi. Eventually, the average length of time it takes to settle into these sixth and seventh limbs will shorten, and the amount of time we are able to stay in them will lengthen, but we may still be moving between all of these states multiple times during one meditation. Figure 4 shows examples of how we might be moving between these states in typical meditation sessions.

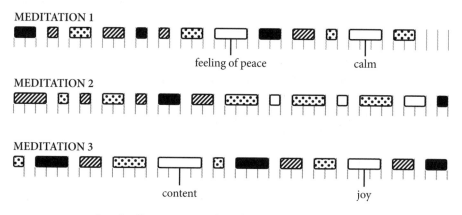

Length of bar represents relative length of time in each state.

■ **External Focus**: on bodily sensations, sensory input, or thoughts of external world

▨ **Internal Focus**: withdrawn from sense or thoughts of external (5th limb/Pratyahara)

▥ **Focus on Meditation Object**: varying degrees (6th limb/Dharana)

☐ **Single-Pointed Focus on Object of Meditation**: may experience pleasant sensations and emotions (7th limb/Dhyana)

Figure 4: Differing Meditation Cycles

It's important to understand these patterns so we don't become discouraged when we don't see clear, linear progression in our meditation. In general, our ability to settle into a new level should strengthen and arise more quickly the more frequently we experience it, but many things can affect this—what is going on in our lives, whether we've been triggered by an external event, our physical health, our ability to practice the preceding limbs. The limbs are sequential but also interdependent, and we may need one more than another at a certain time in our path, depending on what is going on for us. Everyone experiences progress differently; you may find you have many short periods of full concentration interspersed with short periods of distraction. Others may have longer periods of concentration but also longer periods of distraction. Actually mapping this for yourself (the Practice at the end of this section) can help identify ways you may want to tweak your practice.

While we do need to exert effort to progress, it's also important not to relate to the sequential nature of the limbs as a mountain we can *will* or force ourselves to climb. Yogic teachings are very careful to tell us enlightenment isn't something that can be forced. Willpower and discipline are certainly important qualities—part of the second limb—but are not alone what gets us there. Hours and hours of meditation may eventually trigger mystic states but can become a hindrance rather than an aid if we don't process our experiences properly. Developing attachments to these states and neglecting the other limbs actually sets us back. Forcing too much at the concentration level can block us from the seventh and eighth limbs because we are gripping too much in our mind—the equivalent of locking our muscles too rigidly in a balance posture and triggering a fall. Patanjali's advice for the third limb is also relevant here: "*relaxing or loosening effort* allows attention to merge with the infinite." Too much effort can be as much of a problem in meditation as too little.

Practice

- - - - - - - - - - -

CHARTING YOUR MEDITATION CYCLES

- Immediately after each of your next seven meditation sessions, attempt to draw a map along the lines of Figure 4 to depict the periods of time your mind was occupied with thoughts of the outside world, your object of focus, and pure undistracted concentration. Attempt to depict the length of time you spent in each through the length of the line you draw for each period.

- If you experienced feelings like peace or contentment during any of your undistracted phases, note those for yourself as well. While you may not always be able to remember how your meditation progressed, even attempting to do so may help you to become aware of the cycles of your own meditation.

- This information may help you to tweak your practice. Do you see differences based on what you were doing right before you began meditating? Does experimenting with different objects of focus make a difference? Does what you eat or drink beforehand affect it?

- If you experience long periods of distraction, experiment with increasing your level of mental effort/will in order to shorten them—some of the techniques in chapter 2 associated with drowsiness/spaceyness may apply. If you experience a lot of short periods of focus, work with calming methods such as those associated with busyness in chapter 2. Experiment. Meditation is personal, and simply bringing awareness to these cycles may trigger insights.

Seventh Limb—Meditation

Now at last we are at dhyana, meditation. How does Patanjali distinguish between concentration and meditation? One way of understanding it involves imagining thoughts as waves in the mind, each rising and falling just like waves at the beach, one after the other. Some waves are longer and bigger, some are shorter and smaller; sometimes the waves follow one after the other in quick succession, sometimes there are breaks in between. Before yogic practice we don't have much control over these waves in our mind; based on our reactions to what is going on around us, they rise and fall, quicken and slow. Through the first five limbs of yoga we begin to slow and decrease the frequency of these waves by controlling the "weather" that contributes to them: our actions in the world, our internal character, our physical health, and our life force and breath.

Through the sixth limb we begin to work a little differently—by concentrating on an object of focus we attempt to create *one* wave in the mind—a wave so big it overwhelms the others. When we succeed in this, we shift from single-pointed attention (*dharana*) to meditative absorption (*dhyana*). Our mind flows continuously toward our object of focus in one wave. This may last a second or it may last an hour; we may at first go in and out of absorption in small bursts. Eventually we are able to sustain this absorption, or more accurately "rest" in it, because it has the quality of effortlessness. Momentum is created from our concentration, and it is this momentum that carries us into deeper absorption—samadhi, the eighth limb.

One thing meditation is *not* is blankness. It is possible to blank out our mind with our will, to force a single-pointed thought wave of voidness. Although some samadhis are characterized by a realization of the cosmic void, these arise as the sense of self and separateness is released. Constructing a wall of blankness through intense concentration is actually a product *of* self, not a release *from* it. This is one of the ways we can go wrong in yogic meditation—by using our concentration powers to almost mimic a samadhi-like state based on an intellectual understanding of it.

The interplay of dharana and dhyana, concentration and meditation, are where the real heart of yogic spiritual practice lies. Concentration requires will, but too much force keeps us stuck. Dhyana requires letting go, but let go entirely and you'll lose your momentum and slip out of absorption. It's once again about balancing, or "walking the razor's edge," a common metaphor for meditation and the spiritual path in general. Once we find the balance point between will and surrender and can rest there without disruption, we will slip into the eighth limb of samadhi.

Practice
IDENTIFYING CONSTRUCTING VS. CONCENTRATING

• For a few days, after your meditation assess the level of *effort* versus *surrender* within that session. Within effortful phases, did you seek to create or construct a state like blankness? Or was your effort correctly directed at concentrating on your meditative object of focus?

- Constructing versus concentrating feel different in our mind, but it can take time to catch this subtlety. If you sense you may have been putting effort into constructing a state of mind rather than concentrating, experiment with relaxing more *into* your object during periods of focus.

- However, don't overthink it: this kind of assessment (along with the charting from the prior Practice) can be helpful once in a while to help you explore the balance between will/effort and relaxation/surrender. Above all, don't get caught up in this kind of meta-analysis or your practice may become too conceptual. As well, we use our imagination in some practices, so then construction would of course be part of the meditation!

Eighth Limb—The Samadhis

At last, samadhi! Known as "meditative absorption," samadhi is often mentioned in the singular, as though it is one thing, but there are many samadhis. Patanjali names three main types of samadhi, within which are finer divisions. While he does not number them himself, most analysis puts the number at ten samadhis in his system. Some yogic teachings focus only on the broad three types, while others mention hundreds of samadhis we can experience, each as gradations within the larger categories. To some extent, there is a difference because none of these states can really be described in words or concepts. Poetry does it best; indeed, many poems have been written about the experiences of light, joy, peace, stillness, and power available to us in samadhi states. These descriptions are very individual. Describing samadhis in a way that fits a linear model such as Patanjali's is rather difficult.

Patanjali therefore took the approach that is perhaps the most comprehensible—describing types of samadhi in terms of how our mind relates to our object of meditation and to our sense of "I" within each. In the initial samadhis we retain a sense of "I," that we are having an experience, merging with our meditation object, and experience the union that releases waves of peace, joy, and other pleasurable states. As we progress through the samadhis, this identification with "I" is released—the wave of "I" itself in our consciousness settles entirely back into the ocean. We are consumed to a greater and greater degree into our object of meditation until even that dissolves. However, this stage is not spiritual liberation, because we still return to a sense of self after our meditation. The highest level of samadhi is when this merged state is seamless—within both formal meditation and outside of it we know ourselves as both self and Self, wave and ocean, while brushing our teeth, driving our car, or hugging our children.

In the initial samadhis, we merge with our object of meditation through subtler and subtler awareness of it. At first, we are aware of our object's particular qualities, but then gradually this awareness subsides and along with it go the judgments and conceptual ideas *of* that object. At the concentration stage, we may still give attention to particular traits to help us focus—for example, if we picture a deity, we may visualize one body part at a time, or contemplate the qualities or energy associated with that deity in our mind. If we focus on a lit candle, we may notice the colors of the flame or think about the heat produced by fire. But as we move into samadhi, these particular qualities fall away; we move through levels of mind to experience the deity or flame more and more directly. As we do so, our sense of being separate from our object—our sense of "I"—diminishes. These phases of samadhi are sometimes described as having the quality of a "stream of oil being poured"—our mind flows continuously and undistractedly toward our object of meditation, and gradually we are absorbed into it.

In Patanjali's system, this absorption is a category of samadhi called *sabija samadhi*, or "samadhi with seed," that can be experienced at four different levels of consciousness, each of which is itself considered a type of samprajnata samadhi. In addition, the transition state between each of these four is also a samadhi, asamprajnata samadhis, for a total of eight types of sabija samadhi. Some equate these samadhis with salvikalpa samadhi as described in other systems of categorization. The levels of these samadhis are distinguished by the level of "I" waves that still function in the mind—the extent to which you as a meditator still relate to your meditation object as separate from yourself. At first you, the experiencer, the object of your meditation, and the experience itself are still distinct. Your mind is flowing toward your object of meditation in one continuous thought wave, but you retain an awareness of yourself, your object of meditation, and the thought wave connecting you as separate. Gradually, as you move through the samadhis, these distinctions dissolve.

The steps in this process of dissolution are described in various ways by different commentators. One way to understand it is that we first let go of our awareness of the particulars of our object of meditation (as described above). Then we settle into an awareness of the archetype of our object—the concept in our mind of the perfected version of it, which is always present whenever we are focused on a particular. As we let go of this level of mind, we slip into the next level of union with our meditative object, where we are no longer aware of either the object's particulars or its archetype, but rest in a level of mind in which we know the patterns between archetypes. Finally, we let go of even this sense of patterns, and are left with only the object in its wholeness. At this point we have very little of our usual cognitive apparatus functioning, and very little sense of "I." Once this final bit of "I" is released, we settle into the experience of wholeness directly, without a connection to our initial object. Our object of meditation was just a conduit—through merging with it we enter into a wholeness not bound by it. This is samadhi "without seed"—*nibija* or *nirvikalpa* samadhi. When we function from this state in every moment of our lives, we are living in *dharmamegha* samadhi.

Figure 5 shows the samadhis from several different perspectives. The funnel shape of the entire diagram represents the gradual receding of the sense of "I," as represented by the shaded part of each oval level. Every other stage is a new, more abstract, level of merging with our object of meditation—the samprajnata stages. In between these, we experience the transition samadhis of release, the asamprajnata samadhis, as we move beyond one level of awareness of our object and the framework consciousness linked to it, and into another. We finally settle into full union with our object—wholeness. From here, our sense of "I" is entirely dissolved—*nirbija* samadhi. This itself can lead to dharmamegha/kaivalya—on all pervasive knowing of self as Self and all phenomena as self, in and out of meditation.

While it may seem overly conceptual to chart and categorize the meditative journey in this way, it is very in line with the yogic tradition as represented in Patanjali's *Yoga Sutras*. The process is presented as systematic and progressive. While our actual journey rarely progresses in this linear way, these kinds of images and descriptions offer a map for navigation. It's easy to become lost when entering deeper states of meditation; Patanjali's categorizations—and those of later commentaries—are meant to help us avoid this. On the other hand, overintellectualizing the process can become a trap too!

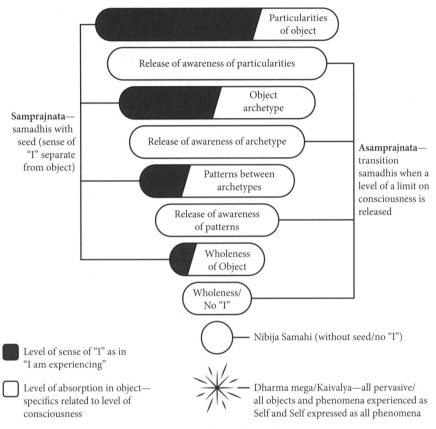

Figure 5: Map of Samadhis

Importantly, in none of these levels of samadhi is there discursive thought as we normally think of it. There may be peripheral or background mental activity in the first samadhis, but we are not identified with it. Discursive thought has already subsided as we slipped from concentration, the seventh limb of dhyana, into samadhi. As we shift between samadhis, the levels we are releasing are conceptual and perceptual frameworks, as well as the structure of a sense of an egoic "I"—frameworks for consciousness as opposed to what we would think of as thoughts. Once discursive thought arises and we identify with it—i.e., "Oh wow, I was just completely absorbed in OM"—we are out of samadhi. We are back to working the limbs of dharana or dhyana. And in fact, limbs six, seven, and eight—concentration, meditation, and samadhi—are together called *samyama*. In any given meditation session, we may be moving back and forth between these three limbs of samyama quite a bit.

While working with samyama, intense emotions and energetic sensations may arise. We may feel intense happiness, relaxation, bliss, or joy. Especially as we experience samadhi, the release of identification can generate experiences at a level of intensity much higher than those released when we experience the peace or calm of extended concentration (*dharana*). At each level we are freed from bonds we didn't know we had, and each release generates powerful surges. If we become attached to these surges, we can become stuck in our search to recreate them each time we sit down to meditate. In fact, we don't move from one level of samadhi to the next until we are done with our current level in Patanjali's yogic system—that is, we must be ready to let go of the experiences to be had there. We let go, let go, let go.

The process of letting go does *and* does not involve our will. Attachment to the experience we are having is one thing that might keep us on a particular plane of samadhi, and the fear of dissolution—of losing our sense of self, of relinquishing our identification as an "I"—is another. Any karmic impressions in our mind or samskaras that keep us tied to our sense of self will also hold us back. It's not uncommon for someone to experience brief periods of samadhi and then not enter them for some time (even lifetimes) due to fears or desires that arise, or karmas that still need to be resolved. At the same time, sitting in samadhi helps cleanse these karmas—we can release them too as we release our sense of self. Time in samadhi can function like a karmic bath, cleansing our being at all its levels of obstructions. But our ability to stay in samadhi long enough for this to occur is based on our practice of all the prior yoga limbs—the fitness and purity of our mind and body.

Nirbija or *nirvikalpa* samadhi is referred to as "without seed" because we have no sense of "I" when in it, no waves of thought towards our object of meditation, and no separation from cosmic consciousness—no duality, only pure awareness and love, the ultimate fruit of union, undifferentiated according to individual beings or objects; beyond time, form, and space. The distinction between subjective and objective reality collapses. Very few ever reach this level; it is associated with the greatest yogis, the greatest spiritual beings of history. Teachings warn us that it's easy to be fooled that we are in this state when in fact we are not—at best, we are in a state of sabija samadhi. My favorite answer to how one would know if they'd been in this state is "you won't care." There's no one there to care.

As wonderful as it may sound, nirbija samadhi is still a state; a meditator will still come out of it at some point. Stories abound of great yogis staying in this state for hours, days, or even weeks at a time. But at some point, they all emerge, just like with sabija samadhi. There is still a sense of meditative reality and everyday reality, and neither is enlightenment within the yogic system. Enlightenment is when cosmic awareness of nibija samadhi is integrated so fully that it is maintained every moment of every day. This is called dharmamegha samadhi, kaivalya, or sahaja samadhi. As unattainable as this state may seem, from a yogic perspective it is our natural state, available to us all. The only thing that blocks us from attaining this state are the impressions of mind formed from holding to past experience, and the sense of a separate self that believes it has had these experiences. As the great spiritual teacher Ramana Maharshi puts it:

> To be one's own Self is Samadhi.
>
> The state, in which awareness is firm, even when the objects are sensed, is called the natural state.
>
> When through practice we are constantly in that state (free from thought—nirvikalpa Samadhi) not going into Samadhi and coming out again, that is sahaja state (the natural state).[35]

Patanjali and every spiritual text on the samadhis emphasize that the experience of them is impossible to put into words. And while Patanjali's descriptions imply ten types of samadhi, the gradations within these in terms of experience are infinite. A more poetic way of describing them is as gradations of light. The clear light of awareness is our natural state, just as white

_ _ _ _ _ _ _ _ _ _ _

35. "Quotes of Sri Ramana Maharshi," Advaita, Ama Yoga, http://elmisattva-nonduality .blogspot.com/2014/10/quotes-of-sri-ramana-maharshi.html.

light is actually all colors of the spectrum combined. Our eyes, however, distinguish many colors; in making those fine distinctions, we discern and label particular gradations. If we look at a color spectrum, the mind latches on to the strong colors—red, orange, yellow, green, and so on. But within and between these is an infinite number of shades—magenta, teal, amber, periwinkle. The possibilities are infinite even though we may be unable to perceive their finer distinctions with our eyes; in other words, the gradations become too subtle.

The same is true of the samadhis: they are gradations of the light of awareness, and as such by definition are infinite. As we tune our awareness through the eight limbs, we are able to experience more of them than we ever imagined possible. We can spend a lot of time enjoying and bathing in these planes of light. But in the end, even this isn't really the purpose of the yogic journey; only when we tire of it can we turn toward complete liberation. We are done with the show, and ready to let go.

Contemplations

Patanjali's eight limbs of yoga are complex, and this chapter covered a lot of material. Even if you do not engage in a yogic form of meditation, see if you can make this material relevant to you through the following questions:

- Do you incorporate some aspect of limbs one through four in Patanjali's yogic system into your life—ethics (first limb), character development (second limb), posture/mind-body modality (third limb), breathing work (fourth limb)? If not, how could you do so? Can you see how they relate to your meditation?

- How do you experience the fifth limb (drawing inward away from sense experience) and sixth limb (concentration)? What do you do inwardly to increase them for yourself? Can you relate to Patanjali's description of concentration as generating one giant thought wave toward your object of meditation?

- Patanajali describes true meditation (the seventh limb) as those times we experience undistracted concentration as one wave in our mind towards our object of meditation. Have you experienced this? Do you regularly move in and out of this in your meditation? What increases your ability to stay in this state for longer?

• Samyama is the interplay between the fifth, sixth, and seventh limbs—drawing inward, concentration, and meditation. How much time do you spend in each in your typical meditation? Can you see how you move in and out of these? What is the relationship between them for you?

• Have you experienced meditative absorption (the eighth limb of samadhi)? How would you describe what you have experienced? How did it come about? Was there still a sense of "I" present? Are you able to let go of this experience, or did your ego grasp on to it?

FIVE

THE BUDDHIST JHANAS

*P**leasure. Joy. Contentment. Stillness. Infinity. Pure Consciousness. The Cosmic Void. Beyond Perception*: these are some of the words used to describe the eight Buddhist jhanas. Like the samadhis, the jhanas are cultivated meditative states; historically the two traditions certainly influenced each other. However, the jhanas are usually described more in terms of how they *feel* to us, how we *experience* them, as opposed to our level of dissolution, and for that reason I find meditators often relate to one or more of them when they first read about them, saying things like "I've experienced that" or "I get that." Some people report having experienced one or more states spontaneously as children, as the Buddha himself is said to have done. While the jhanas are normally taught in a structured, sequential fashion, I believe there is value to reading about them even if you do not plan to pursue them in that manner, as they can help place meditation experiences in a context that helps us to integrate them more deeply.

The teachings on the jhanas are found in some of the earliest Buddhist sutras (oral teachings that were written down) predating Patanjali by two to five hundred years. The jhana teachings are part of Theravada Buddhism, linked to these oldest teachings, as distinct from Buddhist lineages that developed later, including both Zen and Tibetan Buddhism. While these latter two Buddhist traditions don't include jhana teachings exactly like those covered here, the states of meditation referenced in teachings on the jhanas are found both within them and throughout different Buddhist teachings and traditions. The various branches and lineages of Buddhism include many different forms of meditation practice, and some emphasize one or a handful of the jhanic states more than others.

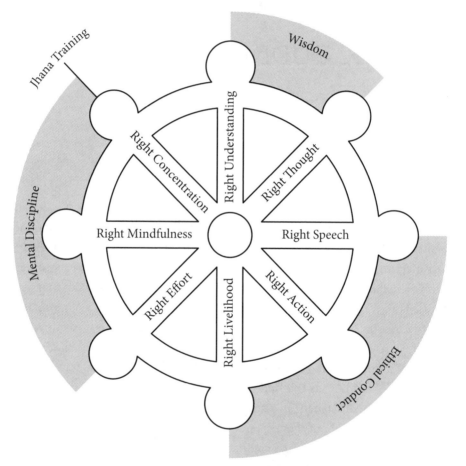

Figure 6: Buddhist Noble Eightfold Path Dharma Wheel

Just as in yoga, meditation within Buddhism cannot be understood apart from the entire Buddhist path. And just as in Patanjali's yoga system, the Buddhist path is also based on eight aspects, together called the Noble Eightfold Path. These components are often presented as eight spokes on a wheel, emphasizing even more their interdependence. All eight components are divided into three divisions: Under Ethical Conduct are Right Speech, Right Action, and Right Livelihood; under Wisdom we find Right Understanding and Right Thought; under Mental Discipline are Right Effort, Right Mindfulness, and Right Concentration. Cultivating the jhanas in meditation falls under Right Concentration but also involves Right Mindfulness and Right View (sometimes called Right Understanding).

Theravada Buddhist traditions differ in their views on the relative importance of developing the jhanas. Some believe insight meditation is more important—insight, or *vipassana* practice begins with mindfulness practice but progresses into subtler direct inquiry into how our mind functions. In some Buddhist traditions, insight is emphasized rather than the jhanas in the belief that it is a more direct path to wisdom. Within insight meditation, we look at our mind in an open and inquisitive way, noting the transience of each thought that arises. Through this process, we discover directly the truth of impermanence (*anitya*), the first step in developing true wisdom. One argument against focusing too much on the jhanas is that we run the risk of increasing our attachment to permanence, our attachment to pleasure, or our attachment to self. And in fact, this is a stated risk of focusing on jhanic states, so teachings include guidance on "correct" and "incorrect" jhana. If we begin to relate to the jhanas purely as a source of pleasure, attachment is created. Likewise, if they become purely mental states (more of an issue in the later or "immaterial" jhanas), and we begin to lose a sense of feeling and emotion, we may find ourselves using the jhanas as a way to disengage or disassociate. Mindfulness is the counterbalancing practice that can help us remain aware of our feelings and sensations, and correct jhana has a quality of mindfulness, and of presence.[36] Jhanic practice also does not exclude insight practice; the concentration we develop through the jhanas gives us the strength of mind to engage in deeper insight meditation and contemplation of teachings. We are more likely to experience new understandings of our mind and how we perceive reality when we engage in inquiry with a stronger mind developed through concentration practice, including jhanic

- - - - - - - - - - - -

36. Gunaratana, *Beyond Mindfulness*, 14.

practice. At the same time, resting in jhanic states helps us release "hindrances" to awakening—habits of mind that block our insight similar to the way the samadhis are taught to release samskaras in Patanjali's path. Mindfulness, concentration, and insight work together in this way.

Bhante Gunaratana in *Beyond Mindfulness in Plain English* emphasizes too the importance of *metta* or lovingkindness practice as part of jhana practice. Metta is a necessary complement to jhana and mindfulness training, because it is through metta we both strengthen our connection with others and release internal blocks or aversions. As a result, we can let go of the attachments to self required to advance in the jhanas:

> When you are flowing metta to all living beings, radiating it outward in all directions with your whole mind...there is simply no room for hindrances. You cannot radiate good will and be greedy at the same time. You cannot be fearful and angry. You cannot have doubts, restlessness, boredom and dullness.[37]

As we progress through the jhanas, the development of our metta is part of what assures we won't grasp our meditation experiences solely for ourselves. Our practice is motivated by a connection to and caring for others, a key component of the Buddhist path, and we stay connected to feeling rather than seek to escape it in some abstract, purely mental, state.

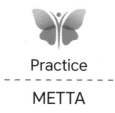

Practice

- - - - - - - - - - -

METTA

- A simple practice of metta involves sending loving thoughts and well-wishes first to yourself and then to wider and wider circles of beings in sequence. You can use statements or visuals to do this, although it's

- - - - - - - - - - - - -

37. Gunaratana, *Beyond Mindfulness*, 59.

more important to cultivate the *feeling* behind the words, so focus on whichever best helps you do this.

- Choose how you want to expand your circle, pausing at each point to really send these feelings out. You may want to visualize your metta going out as light, and beings relaxing or smiling as they receive it.

- You might expand out geographically, or through different types of beings, or just however you feel on a certain day. For example: "I send myself love and well-wishes," "I send my family love and well-wishes," "I send all children love and well-wishes," "I send all animals love and well-wishes," "I send all beings everywhere love and well-wishes."

The First and Second Jhanas—Pleasure and Joy

The first four jhanas are called the "material" or "form" jhanas because they involve feelings we are already somewhat familiar with and that have a tangible quality to them: pleasure, happiness, joy, contentment, tranquility, equanimity. We may have had only brief glimpses of some of these in our lives, but we have some idea of what they are and what they feel like. They are recognizable, although the level and form in which we experience them within the jhanas will likely be new. These jhanas are very motivating—who *doesn't* want to experience these feelings? They feed into the brain's reward cycle mentioned in chapter 2, which is definitely part of their value. Being motivated to practice the jhanas and practice for the length of time it takes to achieve them develops our concentration, which can then be applied to insight practice and the four "immaterial" jhanas—more abstract states that loosen the hold of the ego and contribute more directly to our spiritual awakening.

As with samadhi, a deep level of concentration is necessary to enter the jhanas. Within the sutras are many objects of meditation listed as suitable— our breath, metta, the elements, colored disks used at the time of the Buddha called *kasina,* consciousness itself. Whatever our chosen object of meditation is, absorption with it is the first step. While the jhanas are natural states, in order for us to discover them we have to remove a lot of obstructions. We've already talked about what it takes to get to this point in the last chapter, and the teachings are very similar here—we need to cultivate the proper inner attitude, lifestyle, health, and awareness to enable us to sit down and concentrate. Our preparatory steps clear some of our first level obstructions to discovering our natural states, and our continued vigilance in maintaining these is what will enable us to continue progressing.

As the mind settles, we experience the sensation of sinking into our object of meditation, and with this begin to experience sensations of pleasure and joy. This is our entrance point into the first jhana. We may still have peripheral thoughts and physical pains, but they are now in the background, overwhelmed by the new sensations. We relax into these pleasant feelings and shift our focus away from our object of meditation to the pleasure itself as a feeling in our body. We might focus in on one area of our body where the pleasure feels the most intense and allow it to increase. We then try to sustain this feeling of pleasure and stay in it for a period of time. At first this may only be a few moments, but eventually we will become more adept. The longer we stay in the first jhana, the more intense the energetic sensation of pleasure in the body—rising even to the level of rapture.

With time in the first jhana, we might experience the whole body vibrating with this energy; it can be quite intense. Although different teachers suggest different ways to handle this intensity, as well as different advice regarding how long to stay in this jhana, unless it becomes unpleasant or scary it is considered positive, as time here helps to cut our attachment to worldly pleasures and other hindrances and samskaras. Anyone familiar with kundalini, chakra, or other energy-based meditations will recognize this phenomena. What is interesting about the jhanic path is that although it does not focus upon subtle energies directly, they arise naturally through meditative absorption, especially in this first jhana, and are considered a part of the process.

Some jhana teachers say that we shift naturally into the second jhana when we have spent enough time in the first, and that this is individual to each person, and not something we can dictate. Others say we should consciously try to shift when we feel ready. You may spend many meditation sessions returning to the first jhana, gradually building your ability to get there faster and stay there longer. Being able to repeat it is part of the point; this is not a state of random grace you must wait for. As well, you should be able to find your way back, and with time should be done with it, not get stuck. For most people this happens naturally, as even pleasure gets boring.

A shift into the second jhana is characterized by a feeling of sinking even deeper and settling into the emotion of joy, as opposed to physical sensations of pleasure. Both joy and pleasure are present in the first jhana, but in the second, it is the joy that predominates. This joy has a quality of tranquility to it such that you are no longer filled with the energetic intensity of the first jhana. It feels much more stable and calmer. Any residual mental activity recedes further into the background. There is a quieting, and so to shift into the second jhana you may need to consciously let go of the excitement of the first. The second jhana is refreshing rather than exciting—one metaphor commonly used likens it to a light, gentle rain that cools us on a hot day.

Practice

- - - - - - - - - - -

SHIFTING FROM PHYSICAL TO EMOTIONAL

The principle of shifting between the first and second jhanas by shifting from a physical to an emotional awareness is something you can experiment with in meditation:

- When you experience a physical pleasure or intensity in your meditation, try first focusing *on* and then relaxing *into* the pleasure in your body.

- See if you can gradually relax any excitement or gripping that is accompanying the physical sensations. See if you can settle into the physical sensation without this quality of intensity.

- As you release, settle into a calmer, more tranquil state, and bring your awareness to this as an emotional energy. Relax into it as you would settle into a loved one's hug.

The Third and Fourth Jhanas— Contentment and Stillness

With the third jhana, things get subtler still and our wisdom comes into play. We realize that as wonderful as the first and second jhanas are, they are transient. They come and go, wax and wane. Recognizing this impermanence is a natural outcome of the mindfulness component of jhanic practice and the eightfold path. With this realization we lose interest in joy—we are satiated. We strove and strove to achieve it, but now it is not all that. Through this realization we slide naturally into the third jhana. Some describe this as a feeling of sinking even deeper and suggest consciously relinquishing the joy of the second jhana to help us along. In reality, this relinquishment will not really take, so to speak, until we are truly no longer attached to the joy—that is, achieving a true recognition of its impermanence.

As we sink deeper into the third jhana, we settle into a deep peace and contentment with little to no mental activity, even in the background. In contentment there is no "doing" and very little movement; it is very still. It doesn't have the energetic activity of the first jhana nor the emotional fullness of the second. However, we still retain the feeling of being the experiencer, of experiencing peace and contentment. Our readiness to relinquish this sense of the self as the experiencer is what determines our movement into the fourth jhana. Here's how Theravada Buddhist teacher Ayya Khema describes it in her book, *Visible Here and Now:*

> …[I]f we manage to hold inner peace long enough, it will become increasingly clear that this can't be all there is. With the first three jhanas there was always an observer in place: the ego. But the mind has become more subtle and knows what's what. It sees clearly that peace, joy, and above all the observer have to be abandoned too. Entering the fourth jhana is comparable to sliding into a deep well, where one sinks deeper and deeper. The person whom we know has now willed to give himself or herself up and to sink into this deep well.[38]

Movement into the fourth jhana cannot be rushed. If you attempt to rush it, you run the risk of faking it. The teachings suggest we spend some time perfecting our ability to move in and out of the first three jhanas, figuring out how to enter and sustain them and analyzing why we fall out of them when we do. We will find obstacles of mind—hopes, fears, attachments, and aversions—

---

38. Ayya Khema, *Visible Here and Now: The Buddhist Teachings on the Rewards of Spiritual Practice,* (Shambhala Press, 2001), 110.

that have entered our practice and disrupted our ability to move between the jhanas at will. While we don't want to get stuck in the lower jhanas, mastering these states is instructive and strengthening, and it prepares us for the future jhanas. When we are ready, we relinquish our selves as observers and begin to slide into the fourth jhana. This jhana is characterized by a deep stillness: without the activity of ego, the mind is an absolute still pond on every level. This level is also characterized by light, a luminosity that shines now that we are out of the way. There are many similarities here to how Patanjali describes the samadhis as a progression of dissolution of self/experiencer.

At this point, our meditation practice dovetails with our development of wisdom as the quieting of our ego prepares our mind for deeper insight practice. Nonverbal knowing arises from the fourth jhana, and after we emerge from it is the perfect time to engage in insight practice, inquiring into our own mind, or the contemplation of spiritual texts. Our mind will have unsurpassed clarity and conciseness. We will be able to see truth like never before because the usual mental obstructions are quiet. While at this point in our path these obstructions will likely still return, we can use this time after meditation to deepen our connection to wisdom.

Practice

- - - - - - - - - - -

SCRIPTURAL STUDY

- Explore this relationship between meditation and insight or study by selecting a spiritual text to read excerpts from immediately following your meditation. Even without reaching the fourth jhanic state, you will likely notice how much more clearly you can comprehend material after you have been meditating. With time, this can become your new default level of comprehension and insight; after all, meditation upgrades your brain!

The Fifth and Sixth Jhanas— Limitless Space and Consciousness

With the fifth and sixth jhanas, we enter into the first two of the four immaterial or formless jhanas, which are much more abstract and less linked to the emotions and sensations we recognize from the more mundane side of experience. Although translations vary, the four are roughly known as limitless space, limitless consciousness, voidness, and beyond perception. These are also less connected to our body, which is part of the point. In the first three jhanas we sink into our bodies and the physical and emotional sensations that arise as we focus our meditation and let go of mental constructs; in the fourth jhana we begin to let go of identification with ourselves as the experiencer of either pain or pleasure; in the immaterial jhanas we are at a level of consciousness where our identification with our body is entirely stilled. Within a Buddhist framework, we are motivated to explore the immaterial jhanas because our practice and study shows us that we are truly more than our bodies, that the physical objects of the world are not what they appear, and that identification with the physical world is part of what fuels our suffering.

The immaterial jhanas are understandably very hard to describe in words since there is very little frame of reference for the mind to grasp. And as is hopefully clear, the descriptions of the samadhis and jhanas that appear in this book aren't meant to be full instructions for attaining them; they are offered as a guide to some of the types of experiences that may arise in meditation and how these two traditions place them within the larger context of a spiritual journey. That all said, reading about these states at this level can also be informative…and in some cases a source of relief. Often individuals who have been meditating on their own will have a moment of recognition when they read a description of a jhana or samadhi. The recognition that we and others have experienced some of this before confirms that these experiences are indeed natural and part of our birthright. It also helps us to integrate the experiences and draw wisdom from them.

A recognition of this type occurred for my friend Mike, whom upon first reading about the jhanas, remembered he had frequently experienced the sensation of being in a large empty space within his mind as a young adult. The feeling was disorienting and frightening at the time, and he had blocked out memories of it. As he studied the jhanas more, he realized this state bore many similarities to the fifth jhana of limitless space. He also realized that because this had been fearful to him as a teen, he often held himself back in meditation as an adult due to a subcurrent of anxiety that was always present on the edges of his awareness. As Mike began to settle into more relaxed states, this anxiety would kick into gear and his mind would suddenly become very busy. Realizing that this experience was in fact one cultivated within the jhanas helped him to relax his fear of it, so he could approach his meditation in a more structured fashion that helped him to feel safe.

As with the material jhanas, we move through the immaterial jhanas in sequence by shifting our object of concentration. As we approach the fifth jhana, infinite or limitless space, we are already in a state of great equanimity and stillness where we identify neither with aversion to discomfort nor attraction to pleasure. Various advice is given for how to shift into the fifth jhana, but in essence it boils down to *expansion*: we expand our object of concentration or our sense of our own being out into space, step by step. At first you might expand beyond things you can conceptualize, such as your home, neighborhood, and city. But eventually you must let go even of this and instead focus on a sense of endless expansion.

At some point, a sense of boundless or limitless space will arise. Although you may have worked up to this by focusing on boundless physical space (i.e., going beyond your home, city, and so on), when this space—the fifth jhana—arises, it is not defined by space or of being "beyond" anything else. It is a space within which everything arises, including you. Whether you experience this as something you see or feel is individual. In fact, the space in question is beyond both seeing and feeling, but when you come out of the jhana you need some way to describe it and the mind may grasp one way or another to do so. It's thus important that you don't rely solely on this *memory* to return to the fifth jhana. You want to work with the feeling of expansion until this space naturally arises for you; otherwise, you run the risk of meditation becoming purely conceptual.

As with the other jhanas, traditionally you would learn to stabilize this jhana and enter it at will. Once you have mastered this process, you shift into the sixth jhana, limitless or boundless consciousness. To shift to the sixth jhana, you must have become familiar enough with the fifth jhana to have recognized the sense of the observer, the experiencer, in the space. You bring your attention to the observer or the consciousness aware of the space. Notice that I didn't say "bring your attention to *yourself* observing the space," because if you have traversed through the fourth jhana properly, you already have released your sense of the "I" or separate self who would do the experiencing. The sense of an observer is like a wave or point in the space that you are aware *of* but aren't necessarily identifying *with*. Turn your attention to it, this consciousness, and from there realize the limitlessness of this consciousness itself. Leigh Brasington, author of *Right Concentration* puts it this way:

> The trick for moving to the sixth jhana is to shift your attention from the space to your consciousness of the space. Become aware of your awareness; become conscious of your consciousness. It's a trick of turning your mind back on yourself. Since you can't be conscious of the limitless space with a limited consciousness, when you turn your attention back to your consciousness, lo and behold, it's as big as the limitless space, and you are now aware of having limitless consciousness.[39]

These states can be very trippy, but it's still possible to relate to them in a way that is egocentric or dissociative (we'll discuss traps such as this in relation to all forms of meditation in chapter 8). If you are really in the fifth or sixth jhana you would not describe it as you yourself experiencing limitless space or limitless consciousness; instead it is as if the experience of *you* arises within limitless space or consciousness. It is a total shift in orientation. The difference, again, is whether you have mastered the fourth jhana and whether you have processed your experience from the perspective of releasing the "I-ness."

The Seventh and Eighth Jhanas— Voidness and Beyond Perception

The seventh jhana is alternately translated as voidness, the sphere of no-thingness, or the base of nothingness. Some meditation traditions make mention of "the void," and as covered in the last chapter, we may be prone to mimic this state by mentally creating and focusing on a *concept* of vast emptiness because of this term. The jhanas are not conceptual, however; in order to ensure we are not engaging in this kind of conceptualization, we enter this

- - - - - - - - - - - -

39. Leigh Brasington, *Right Concentration: A Practical Guide to the Jhanas*, (Boston: Shambhala Press, 2015), 79.

jhana only after the prior jhanas. In the fifth jhana, we focused on expansion until limitless (nonconceptual!) space arose for us, and in the sixth we turned our focus to the consciousness aware of this space—awareness of awareness. To shift into the seventh jhana, we turn our attention to another aspect of the limitless space: its lack of content or objects. There is nothing (that is, "no thing") in the space, anywhere we may look—this includes mental objects of thoughts, ideas, or archetypes. The shift from the awareness of the space (fifth jhana) to the awareness of the nothing-ness (seventh jhana) is a shift in orientation, and it comes through an additional sense of expansion.

Like limitless space, voidness can be disorienting if we are plunged into it with no preparation or way to process it, something that sometimes happens to beginner meditators or as the result of mind-altering substances. Part of the purpose of jhana training is to create a container and structure for these kinds of explorations, wherein this jhana actually feels free of its baggage, something like relief. Nobody wants anything from us, there is nothing here to scare us, we are free of our usual limiting mind states. However, we still are perceiving, having a sense of ourselves as perceiving objectlessness, just like there was the sense of perceiving space in the fifth jhana and perceiving consciousness in the sixth. The eighth and final jhana is about moving beyond even this perception into neither perception *nor* non-perception.

Describing perception requires identifying and labeling, so the eighth jhana is even harder to describe because there are no identifying characteristics or labels to use. In the first four jhanas we could reference sensations and feeling; in the fifth through seventh we could reference space, consciousness, and nothingness. Even though as you read this you are relating conceptually, you are still allowed a glimpse into what these as non-conceptual experiences might be. But the description "neither perception nor non-perception" does not have these signposts. Instructions for shifting into the eighth jhana are also hard to convey; some teachers suggest there is no step for doing so, that it simply happens when one has released all the hindrances and attachments to other states. There is a common theme of collapse, as in the collapse of the voidness of the seventh jhana, as well as a collapse of your entire perceptual framework along with it.

Although it's tempting to equate this eighth jhana with the dissolution of "I" (equivalent to Patanjali's nibija samadhi "without seed"), it is not characterized as such in Buddhist teachings. All jhanas are states we can train ourselves to move in and out of—they are transient, and the subtle identification with "I" as experiencer remains. However, at each level this becomes fainter, and the release of identification with our sensations, emotions, and the body must go in order to enter the immaterial jhanas prepares us for the deeper realizations that precede awakening on the Buddhist path. Awakening is not something we move in and out of, not a state we enter at will, but instead a realization or recognition, of the nature of reality. Jhana training is meant to support this realization, not become a meditation trick we can do or experience we can have for its own sake.

Like the samadhis, the jhanas provide a map for our meditation journey. Not everyone progresses in this linear way, but there's often value in looking at a practice within the context of a different map. Figure 7 provides one look at the jhanas to close out our exploration of them. Rather than show the jhanas as a ladder, I've chosen to show them in a horseshoe shape, because the first four material jhanas all have the characteristic of sinking deeper as we move through them. The transition between each of these states involves quieting another aspect of our mind—first physical, then emotional, then of experience itself. At the fourth jhana, we might choose to use the clarity of mind that arises from our deep stillness for insight practice or study, or we might focus on expansion to shift into the fifth jhana of limitless space. To rise through the immaterial jhanas, we open wider as more abstract frameworks for consciousness are experienced and then released.

Practice

- - - - - - - - - -

MAPPING YOUR PATH

- Maybe you are engaged in a spiritual path with a different map, or maybe you have your own. If so, draw it for yourself: what have been your seminal experiences and insights? What triggered the transition from one state to the next? Creating a visual map for yourself like this can help you get a sense of what your next frontier may be.

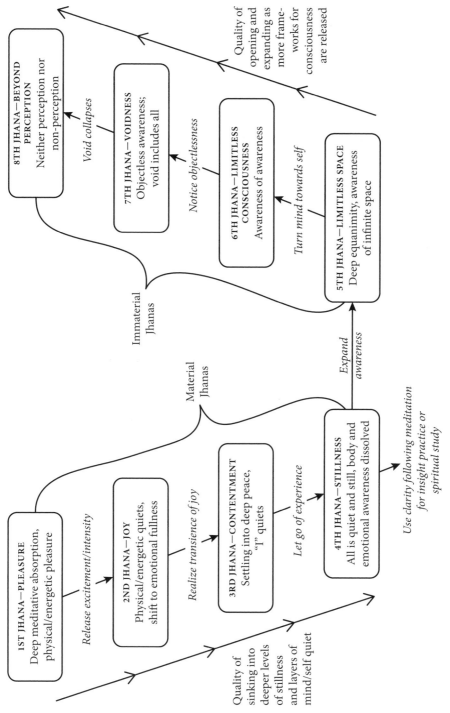

Figure 7: Jhanas Map

Contemplations

- Do you relate more to descriptions of the samadhis or the jhanas? Do you feel you have experienced some of the jhanas? If so, which ones?

- Regardless of whether you study in a Buddhist tradition, what is your understanding of the idea that meditation fuels insight and wisdom when we are "off the cushion"? Can you think of times meditation has fueled your ability to understand a spiritual truth or your own self-awareness?

- Do you relate more to descriptions of the immaterial or immaterial jhanas? Why do you think that is? Can you enter any at will? Are you attached to any of these states?

- How have your sense of self and your experience as an "I" changed through meditation? How has it reshaped your ideas about your own consciousness?

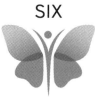

SIX

OTHER MAPS OF THE SEEKER'S JOURNEY

Both the yogic and jhana traditions begin with concentration on a mental object or anchor, but not all forms of meditation do. In insight meditation, we examine reality and our own consciousness as we contemplate a particular question or aspect of mind. Just as with concentration practice, there are insight stages we may progress through that involve personal inquiry into subtler and subtler layers of mind and our perception of reality. Some lineages of Zen Buddhism focus on the contemplation of *kōan*, questions that have no rational answer, the most famous example of which is "What is the sound of one hand clapping?" The process of contemplation in this manner leads not to an answer that logic or the mind can accept but to an exploration and collapse of conditioned mental frameworks, which provides a glimpse of the awakened mind.

Other traditions contemplate spiritual texts, poetry, and even sacred music. Some incorporate movement meditations, from walking mindfulness to the spinning dervish dance. While I personally believe there's a lot of value in understanding the role of meditation across multiple traditions, it's important not to conflate them all. Details matter, and in order to progress spiritually (if that's your aim), it's important to commit to a path and dig deep. If you are already digging deep, the value of surveying other traditions is to gain perspective on your own. To that end, this chapter briefly covers how a few more traditions conceptualize the contemplative journey. These particular traditions have been chosen because I believe they each have something of relevance for the modern practitioner:

- **Kundalini Rising:** Understanding of how meditation triggers releases and shifts in our energy body
- **Ancient Egyptian Mysticism:** Exploring the power of symbolism
- **Kabbalah:** Understanding the link between esotericism and layers of mind
- **St. Teresa of Avila's Interior Castle:** Viewing the spiritual path as progressive intimacy with God
- **Sufism:** Divine love as a path to divine union

Through the Practices and Contemplations are ways you can experiment with these particular aspects of these traditions.

Kundalini Rising

Though Sara was not a spiritual seeker, in her late twenties she began experiencing powerful surges of energy that kept her up at night. Having just gone through a divorce, she at first chalked up her experiences to anxiety and sought medication from her doctor. However, the surges did not stop, and at times she would also see planes of colored light and unfamiliar symbols in her mind when she closed her eyes. She sometimes experienced intense heat or a tingling in her forehead. Her tastes in food began to change, and her sensitivity to light and sound increased. After multiple consultations with doctors, none of whom could find anything wrong, Sara finally came across information online that seemed to be describing her symptoms exactly: a kundalini awakening. Sara found a yoga center that taught kundalini meditation and with instruction, her symptoms began stabilizing and receding almost immediately. These experiences led Sara to embark on a deep spiritual path that included a regular meditation practice that continues to this day.

I met Sara much later in her journey but have heard many stories like hers over the years. *Kundalini* is the Sanskrit term for "spiritual energy," or the energy of consciousness that underlies our subtle body and activates as part of our spiritual journey. Some yogic and Buddhist traditions work with it exclusively: kundalini yoga, kundalini meditation, chakra meditation, kriya yoga, and other energy-based spiritual practices all employ methods for strengthening and directing this energy to facilitate spiritual awakening. However, any personal or spiritual growth involves some kind of kundalini shift; it is not these traditions exclusively that activate it. Many of the energetic sensations associated with the samadhis and jhanas, mystic states of saints from other religious traditions, and visionary states from various shamanic traditions are clearly activations of the kundalini. What is unique about kundalini-based traditions is that they work to trigger this energy *directly,* not as a byproduct of other practices. Kundalini work is sometimes described as an energy technology in this way—a tool for facilitating the spiritual journey.

When triggered through meditation or yoga practice, kundalini shifts are rarely as uncomfortable as what Sara experienced. In fact, the states of pleasure and peace associated with our mind settling for brief periods in beginning meditation are associated with the first gentle waves of the kundalini rising. However, spontaneous kundalini shifts like the ones she experienced do sometimes occur and are often linked to major life events (in her case a divorce). In those cases, working explicitly with kundalini and chakra-based practices—or with an energy worker or therapist in extreme cases—can help ground and stabilize the energy surges.

The roots of kundalini teachings are as old as yoga itself, which is to say, older than we really know, because even in Patanjali's time, yoga had been around for quite a while. Like all yoga traditions, it has been codified and developed by various teachers over the centuries, and we now have many different lineages and organizations actively teaching it. Although there is overlap, each tends to have its own specific practices and maps for progression. One of the most well-known kundalini meditation programs in the West is structured around twenty-one progressive stages. Paramahansa Yogananda, one of the first Indian teachers to bring yogic teachings to the West and founder of the Self-Realization fellowship, divided his Kriya Yoga path into six main stages with smaller sub-stages within each. In general, formal kundalini paths such as these require the initiation and guidance of a teacher.

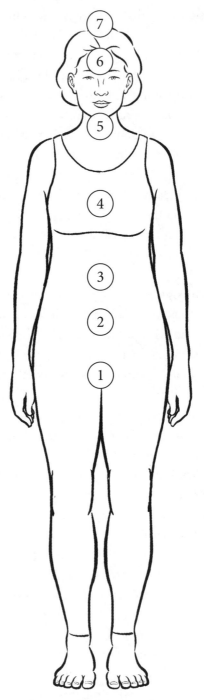

Figure 8: Chakra Access Points

Because each kundalini-based path has specific exercises and stages, there isn't one progression that can be summarized here. That said, a common way of looking at kundalini-based paths in the modern day is through the lens of the chakras and the psychological functions and aspects of consciousness associated with each. Chakras are nexuses of energy that the kundalini energy travels through as part of the awakening process to loosen karmic obstructions (among other things), and many kundalini practices involve consciously bringing the kundalini energy into one or more chakras individually or in sequence. While chakras are referenced in most (if not all) kundalini-based traditions, they don't all use the same chakra mappings. For that matter, it is not only kundalini-based traditions that have energy center mappings like the chakras; many spiritual and energy healing traditions all around the world do.[40] Figure 8 shows the seven chakra focal points I like to use, as part of the seven-chakra system most commonly known in the West.

The awakening process from a kundalini perspective involves the movement of the kundalini energy from its base at the first (or root) chakra, associated with the base of the spine, through all the chakras to the top chakra at the crown of the head. However, this root-to-crown model is not viewed exactly literally or linearly in every tradition; a particular individual's kundalini may be mostly congregated in a chakra other than their root, or it may be particularly active or blocked in one or more chakras, all depending on a person's energy body's karmic level. Women's energy bodies tend to be oriented around the sacral chakra, located in the pelvic bowl, and the access point for this chakra differs for men and women, just as our reproductive organs—linked to the sacral chakra—differ.[41] In other words, the root to crown journey of the kundalini is a generalized, big-picture model for looking at spiritual progression energetically, but most of us do not literally progress from one chakra to the next in this way.

Kundalini may be active within a chakra at varying levels. If we meditate on a specific chakra by holding focus there or we are working through a block associated with a chakra, we may experience sensations or states of

- - - - - - - - - - - -

40. For a look at chakra mappings from all around the world, see Cyndi Dale's *Llewellyn's Complete Book of Chakras,* listed in the Recommended Book List.

41. For more information on women's energy bodies, please reference my own book *Chakra Empowerment for Women* listed in the Recommended Book List.

awareness linked to the vibration and opening of that chakra. We might also be in a phase of our life (or entire incarnation!) in which obstructions as they are expressed at the energy body level "hold" our kundalini in one or more chakras, and our life experience reflects the themes and energies associated with them more prominently than others. Both levels may be functioning simultaneously—for example, we may have strong heart chakra experiences during meditation but more generally in life are working through sacral chakra issues, or vice versa.

What follows are examples of the life themes often associated with the chakras in contemporary writings on them, along with the meditative states or sensations associated with each chakra's opening. These do vary somewhat by tradition, and to some extent have been developed in more recent times through the influence of modern psychology (you won't find a list like this in the *Yoga Sutras*!). The general idea is that if we are in a phase of life in which we are processing karmas related to a chakra, it will reflect that chakra's themes in our life experiences. If we are experiencing energy shifts related to a particular chakra, that may also reflect in certain kinds of spiritual experiences related to that chakra, or even physical sensations near that chakra.

Root Chakra/First
- **Life Themes:** Safety, security, connection to ancestry, grounding, physicality, relationship to body, relationship to material world (including money)
- **Experiences of Opening:** Feeling fully present, physically "in the zone," deep connection to nature/earth, fully embodied

Sacral Chakra/Second
- **Life Themes:** Inspiration, emotion, pleasure, sensuality, sexuality, feminine energy
- **Experiences of Opening:** Bodily pleasure as spiritual, "muse" creative energy (sense of receiving an idea), divine or archetypal feminine, embodied joy, sacred sexuality

Navel Chakra/Third
- **Life Themes:** Will, power, self-definition, self-esteem, organization, boundaries, energy levels
- **Experiences of Opening:** Interdependence/connection to all things, wholeness, vitality, intent as conduit for spiritual forces (not personal/egoic), deep concentration (absorption)

Heart Chakra/Fourth
- **Life Themes:** Relationships, tolerance, self-acceptance, compassion, balance
- **Experiences of Opening:** Universal love, unconditional compassion, merging with the divine, spontaneous healing

Throat Chakra/Fifth
- **Life Themes:** Communication, honesty, authenticity, self-presentation
- **Experiences of Opening:** Merging with vibration (might be mantra, music, or any other sound), body as vibrational bliss, equanimity

Third Eye Chakra/Sixth
- **Life Themes:** Vision, intuition, insight, dreaming, imagination
- **Experiences of Opening:** Mystic visions, deep stillness, boundarylessness, timelessness, epiphany

Crown Chakra/Seventh
- **Life Themes:** Trust, faith, sense of purpose, meaning, spiritual connection
- **Experiences of Opening:** Light, surrender, release of self, divine union, nonduality

While this is a very basic map, it gives some idea of how you might look at your spiritual journey from the perspective of the chakras. We may spiral through all of these phases and experiences many times in the course of a lifetime (or lifetimes), each time opening on a deeper level. Within a structured kundalini path, specific exercises are designed to open one or more chakras and may trigger the associated opening experiences that, similar to the samadhis or jhanas, are not the end goal but helpful steps along the way. Psychological balance and insight are key in order to process energetic shifts as they occur.

Kundalini paths include a lot of warnings about raising the kundalini in a paced and measured way under the direction of a teacher or mentor. If the kundalini is activated too quickly or a person is not stable enough to process it, physical and mental imbalances can result. Sometimes called "kundalini crises," these sudden bursts of kundalini activity are often preceded by a life-changing event (as in Sara's case) or a major astrological transit and may require the help of an energy-aware therapist, intuitive, or healer to work through. The integration process typically first involves stabilizing and grounding the energy through root chakra work, followed by smoothing the flow of the activated energy, and then working from a counseling perspective to understand the psychological impact and roots of the experience in order to process it psychologically. Fortunately, these kinds of experiences are relatively rare. We will talk more about energy disturbances and how to handle them in meditation in Chapter 8.

Practice

CHAKRA MEDITATION

- If you would like to experiment with chakra meditation, the best chakra to focus on without formal training is the heart chakra. As the center point in virtually any chakra system, focusing here contributes to overall energetic balance and equanimity. There are different ways to connect with the chakras—the most common are visually, kinesthetically, or emotionally. You can pick one or all three as the anchor for your meditation.

- To experiment with visual accessing, simply imagine a radiant white sphere of light in the center of your chest, beneath the midpoint of your breastbone.

- To experiment with physical accessing, press gently onto your breastbone and use the physical sensation as the anchor for your focus.

- To try emotional accessing, think of someone you love and see if you feel a warmth in your mid-chest area—if so, let go of your thought and focus on the warm feeling as your meditation object.

- Use the white sphere, the physical contact, or the warm feeling as the focus point of your meditation, returning to it again and again, deepening the connection, and sit for as long as you like.

Ancient Egyptian Book of Coming Forth by Day

"Not a perfect soul, I am perfecting. Not a human being, I am a human becoming."[42] One of my favorite lines from Normandie Ellis's beautiful *Awakening Osiris: A New Translation of the Egyptian Book of the Dead* captures her reading of this ancient Egyptian text as a map for the spiritual journey. Although commonly known as the *Egyptian Book of the Dead,* this set of scrolls is more properly translated as the *Book of Coming Forth by Day* and is largely considered a funerary text that was placed in tombs with the deceased to aid them on their journey through the afterlife. However, some consider the work to be a metaphorical guide to the spiritual journey while alive, a journeying into spiritual light and rebirth.

The most well-known version of this text, the Papyrus of Ani, housed in the British Museum, depicts the stages of the *ba* (one part of the soul as ancient Egyptians considered it) traversing the pathway to the afterlife. Those who read the Papyrus of Ani as a map for the enlightenment process see in each step a symbol for a level of awakening. Portrayed through exquisite images and hieroglyphics (themselves image-based), an analysis of these images can show the power of symbolism to portray multiple levels of meaning. Many of these levels are found throughout different mystic traditions, all of which point to a universal spiritual process:

- **Descent into the Underworld:** The ba's descent into the underworld represents the conscious decision to turn away from conditioned existence, embark on the spiritual journey, and look at its full self—the shadows or subconscious—in an effort to be liberated from it/them. In the context

--- --- --- --- --- --- --- --- --- --- --- --

42. Normandi Ellis, *Awakening Osiris: A New Translation of the Egyptian Book of the Dead,* (Grand Rapids, MI: Phanes Press, 2009), 25.

of meditation, this involves practices that focus on surfacing and working through obstructive patterns, limiting self-perceptions, and worldly attachments.

- **Slaying of Monsters:** As the ba travels through the underworld, it is confronted by many terrifying and manipulative creatures, all of whom try to stop its progress. These represent the many personal demons and challenges we face in our spiritual growth. In the context of meditation, these obstacles represent our own fears, projections, distractions, and traps that potentially stall us and that we must work through.

- **Waiting in Line:** Eventually the ba reaches the Hall of Ma'at, or Hall of Judgment, where it must wait in line with many others. This waiting represents the long phase of patient practice and moral purification required to prepare the soul for wisdom, and eventually ascent.

- **Facing of the Forty-two Judges:** The ba faces forty-two judges one by one, and declares to each it has not committed a particular moral offense, i.e., "I have not lied," or "I have not stolen." Each judge must allow passage for the soul to continue. Interestingly, a scarab placed over the deceased's heart was said to protect it from betraying any lapse that may have occurred. This process can be seen to represent the soul's moral purity, and the scarab the recognition and atonement for any past transgressions—as long as personal responsibility has been taken, the transgression has been purified. Meditatively, this phase represents the purification and shifts that occur in the various levels of consciousness traversed in meditation.

- **Weighing of Heart:** The heart of the deceased is now weighed against the feather of Ma'at, which represents truth, justice, and righteousness. If the heart is heavier than the feather, the soul is obliterated. If it is as light as a feather, it begins its ascension, or begins experiencing the higher vibrations of light.

- **Travel Across the Lake of Lilies:** In order to reach the paradisal field of reeds, the ba must successfully navigate the beautiful lake of the lilies. Meditatively, this step could be compared to navigating the samadhis, i.e., not getting caught in their blisses but seeing through to the full reality of awakening.

- **Field of Reeds:** The ba's final destination is a life just like it had before—the same home, family, and activities, but without suffering. Here the ba lives for all eternity. Like the Zen phrase "before enlightenment chop wood and carry water, after enlightenment chop wood and carry water," the end game is not a magical realm or new life, but waking up—that is, coming forth by day in the life we have.

Many traditions contain texts that can be read on either an exoteric or esoteric level, and meditation in most is considered part of the esoteric path. Symbols are the heart of esoteric readings, such as in this interpretation, where the images of descension, monsters, the weighing, the lake, the field of reeds, and more are all read metaphorically. Symbols speak directly to our unconscious, relaying meaning and knowledge beyond words. Many meditation traditions in fact use symbols as meditation objects—yantras, mandalas, deities, and sacred art. Layered meaning, and esoteric interpretation, is at the heart of the next three traditions we'll look at as well.

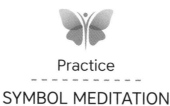

Practice

- - - - - - - - - - - -

SYMBOL MEDITATION

You can experiment with using a symbol as your meditation object through either symbol gazing or visualization.

- Select a spiritual symbol that has meaning to you, and whose qualities or significance you would like to cultivate more of within your own consciousness.

- To meditate on this symbol, you can either gaze at an image of it with relaxed vision or close your eyes and visualize the symbol before you in your mind's eye.

• Focus on the particular attributes of the symbol at first, but relax into a more abstract connection as your focus increases. Allow the symbol to settle into all layers of your psyche. Allow yourself to absorb it on a nonconceptual level.

Sefirot of Kabbalah

Kabbalah is often referred to as Jewish Mysticism, although there were Christian and Hermetic Kabbalah traditions that developed at various points in history that are reflected today within Western Theosophy and other Western esoteric traditions. Kabbalah is comprised of esoteric teachings on the infinite, unknowable aspect of God and all creation—the finite, knowable world. Formal Kabbalah study within orthodox Judaism involves intense scriptural and theological study in addition to contemplative practices and is reserved for only the most serious. As Kabbalah practices have become more known, other Jewish spiritual leaders have begun to incorporate forms of Jewish meditation that originated in Kabbalah into teachings for a broader spectrum of people.

Many of these forms of meditation are similar to yogic and Buddhist practices in that they incorporate mantras, visualizations, and a system of energy centers within the body. While some have used this as an argument against their use in the opinion that they are a co-mingling and therefore corruption of spiritual systems, Aryah Kaplan, a foremost orthodox Jewish writer on Kabbalah argues that the similarities in such practices across traditions actually validates their effectiveness rather than undermines their legitimacy. He points out that every religion uses prayer and worship as well, noting:

> This does not make Jewish worship and prayer any less meaningful or unique, and the same is true of meditation. It is basically a technique for releasing oneself from the bonds of one's physical nature. Where one goes from there depends very much on the system used.[43]

---

43. Aryan Kaplan, *Meditation and Kabbalah,* (San Francisco: Weiser, 1986), 3.

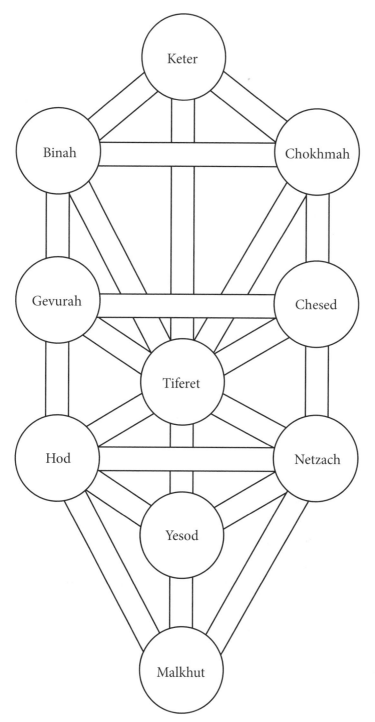

Figure 9: Kabbalah Tree of Life

Within Kabbalah, the primary model for understanding the relationship between the infinite/unknowable and finite/knowable forms of God is through the ten *sefirot* (or *sephiroth*). Each *sefirah* is considered a different divine emanation and is associated with a different name of God, vowel sounds, energies active in the world, and aspects of the psyche. Through both study and meditation practices, the Kabbalah student comes to know God through understanding and experiences of these different aspects. In this way, the ten sefirot serve as both a model for spiritual study and as a way of categorizing spiritual experience. They are traditionally depicted in a ladder-like structure of interconnected nodes called the Tree of Life, with some sefirot located on the right, representing their masculine nature; others located on the left, representing the feminine; and the rest in the middle, representing union. From top to bottom, the Tree of Life represents God's creation; from bottom to top, it represents our pathway to knowing God through creation.

Like all the esoteric traditions, Kabbalah is vast and complex, so what follows here is just a brief overview of the ten sefirot from the perspective of how they map to the spiritual path and meditation experiences as reflections of aspects of the divine.

- **Keter:** "Crown." That which is above and beyond the mind's comprehension. God as infinite, unknowable, and beyond any analysis or description. Associated with humility and purity on the spiritual journey, as this is our proper orientation to God.
- **Chokhmah:** Wisdom and insight that are realized or inspired, not stemming from rationality. Associated with the experience of light and flashes of spiritual insight or epiphany.
- **Binah:** Understanding and processed wisdom—taking the realizations of Chokhmah and applying them using rationality and life experience. Also associated with repentance, as acknowledgment of wrongdoing is the first step in atoning for it.
- **Da'at:** Central mystical state where all ten sefirot meet and are realized as one (therefore not technically itself a sefirah). It is not always shown

in depictions of the Tree of Life, as it is the meeting point of all the sefirot as opposed to being a sefirot itself.

- **Chesed:** Kindness and love, the first of the emotion-based sefirot. It is the foundation for charity and good works in the world, and in terms of meditation is associated with experiences of receiving divine love and emanating compassion.

- **Gevura:** Limits and judgment of right and wrong. It complements the outward unconditional impulse of Chesed with rules and accountability. Meditatively, it is associated with discernment and discipline.

- **Tiferet:** Compassion, beauty, and balance—this is where Chesed and Gevura come together balancing love and discipline. Connected to all the sefiroth except the top, Keter, and bottom, Malkhut, this represents the central work of the spiritual journey, including the actual practice of meditation—the balance of giving (Chesed) and receiving (Gevura) divine energies.

- **Netzach:** Timelessness, eternity, and endurance. It represents the patience and commitment in relation to spiritual practice, as well as pushing through obstacles and the experience of timelessness.

- **Hod:** Transcendence and sublimity, linked to prayer. Netzach and Hod complement each other, as Netzach has a quality of pushing through obstacles, while Hod has a quality of surrender.

- **Yesod:** Connection, action, and energy. It represents the balance of Netzach and Hod, and in meditation this reflects as the balance between pushing through and surrender. Yesod is also the interface between all the other sefirot and the world as represented by Malkhut and is therefore also linked to sexuality and creation. Meditatively, in this aspect it represents union of the masculine and feminine, and embodied bliss.

- **Malkhut:** Physical/seen world, matter, emanating from creation. The densest and "furthest" from Keter, but also containing the seeds from within which all sephirot may be realized. In terms of meditation, Malkhut represents mindfulness, especially mindfulness of body—our vehicle for all spiritual practice.

While metaphorically the Tree of Life represents the journey from the material world to God from bottom to top, in practice this process doesn't unfold linearly—a seeker works all of the sefirot at the level they are capable of within both formal spiritual practice and daily life. The Tree of Life portrays an integrated spiritual path in addition to providing a map of creation. This is true of many traditions' spiritual maps—they reflect a theology as well as a journey, and the levels of the universe as represented within the cosmic theology are also experienced directly beyond words—and the intellectual mind—by way of meditation.

Practice

- - - - - - - - - - -

SCRIPTURAL MEDITATION

- Kabbalah values contemplative scriptural study as a means for esoteric understanding and realizations. Many traditions have a variation on this kind of practice, including *lectio divina* ("divine reading") in Christianity. You can explore this by centering your meditation around an important phrase or paragraph from a sacred text important to you.

- Repeat the phrase or read the paragraph several times at the start of your meditation and allow your mind to quiet.

- Repeat the phrase or reading each time discursive mind returns.

- Do this for as long as you like and then journal afterward on your understanding of your phrase or reading.

St. Teresa of Avila's Interior Castle

Esoteric and symbolic presentations of the spiritual journey exist within the many branches of contemplative Christianity as well, and one of the most well-known and profound is that presented by Saint Teresa of Avila in her *Interior Castles* (or *The Mansions*). Presented as seven stages of the soul's progression from "sin to the Bride of Christ," Saint Teresa describes her metaphor this way:

> I began to think of the soul as if it were a castle made of a single diamond or of very clear crystal, in which there are many rooms, just as in heaven there are many mansions...some above, others below, others at each side; and in the center and midst of them all is the chiefest mansion where the most secret things pass between God and the soul.[44]

Teresa's vision presents the journey to God as one of increased intimacy—we move step by step toward the heart of the castle, where the closest relationship is available to us. We begin outside all seven mansions; to even enter, prayer and deep humility are required. The First Mansion, the Mansion of Humility, is surrounded by dangerous creatures that represent the temptations to sin in the world. It is only by dwelling here and resisting them for some time that the soul becomes qualified to enter the Second Mansion. Surviving these creatures is not simply a matter of discipline but of even deeper humility than was required to enter in the first place. For Saint Teresa, humility was synonymous with a greater awareness of one's smallness in the face of God, and of God's infinite goodness and love. As our soul turns toward this goodness and away from sin, we gradually become capable of receiving streams of God's love, creating an even greater capacity for humility.

When our soul has been purified through humility within the First Mansion, we progress to the Second Mansion, of the Practice of Prayer. Though we are still at risk from the outside creatures of sin, through prayer our soul's humility and faith are fortified yet more, until we are ready to move deeper inward, to the Third Mansion, of Exemplary Life. In this stage, our soul is strong and less susceptible to outside forces, possessing both the capacity for charity and discipline. The danger, however, is now egoism—viewing these strengths as our own rather than as gifts from God. It is only once this egoism is released that our soul may enter the Fourth Mansion, the Mansion of the Prayer of the Quiet.

- - - - - - - - - - -

44. St. Teresa of Avila translated by Mirabai Starr, *The Interior Castle*, (New York: Riverhead Books, 2004), 19–20.

The first three mansions are considered external, concerned with the outside world. The remaining mansions are purely interior, traversed through meditation and contemplation. In the Fourth Mansion, our soul turns entirely toward God and is capable of receiving God's love like water from a never-ending fountain. Attachments to the outside world are sundered, as the soul wants only to continue on its path to Union. In the Fifth Mansion, the Prayer of Union, the soul experiences even deeper absorption to the point of complete possession by God, although our souls are only able to sustain this for short periods.

In the Sixth Mansion, the Mansion of the Bride and Groom, this absorption or possession lasts for longer periods of time. The Bride is our soul, and the Groom is Christ as Christ-consciousness—the experience of the aspect of God that can be met by the soul. This Mansion is also associated with tests such as sickness, depression, persecution, and other challenges. In order to progress to the Seventh (and innermost) mansion, we must hold steady in our devotion through it all. Only once we have succeeded do we enter the Seventh Mansion of Spiritual Marriage—complete Union with God through Christ, something Saint Teresa likened to "another heaven."

Sufi Maqamat

The spiritual journey as one of devotional union with the divine is also the heart of the Islamic mystic branch of Sufism. The devotional poems of thirteenth-century Sufi mystic and poet Rumi are treasured throughout the world for their portrayal of divine love between himself and his "Beloved." Sufi spiritual practices revolve around cultivating and expressing the ecstasy that arises from the experience of this love by way of meditation, poetry, music, and most famously dancing, in the form of whirling dervishes, from the Mevlevi Order of Sufism. In addition to writing poetry, Rumi was also a teacher who wrote prose on the Sufi spiritual awakening process. In these writings, he described the process in devotional terms *and* as the death of the ego:

> In God's presence, there is no room for two egos. You say
> "ego," and he says "ego"? Either you die in his presence, or
> he will in your presence, so that no duality may remain. Yet
> it is impossible that he should die either in the universe or in

the mind, for "He is the living, who does not die." (Qur'an 25:58). He has grace in such measure that, were it possible, he would die for you to remove the duality. But since his death is impossible, you die, so that he may become manifest in you and the duality be lifted.[45]

Within Sufism, the meditation practice of *muraqabah* ("to observe") aids the seeker in moving through the levels of *nafs* or states of being that block a seeker from knowing themselves as Allah. The lower states are purely egoic, with the soul identifying only with the world and people in it, alternately blaming others and the self for suffering. Eventually, the soul progresses to subtler and subtler nafs; in each, the veil of separation from the divine becomes thinner until at last we are prepared for union. Although there are many Sufi lineages, and not all describe the same states of meditation along this journey, a conventional map presents the process as one of progressing from *ghanood*, "somnolence," to *baqaa*, "eternal union."

Within this model, as a meditator we first experience meditation as somnolence or sleep; that is, the literal drowsiness one may experience while practicing in addition to the metaphorical "sleep" or the state of separation from the divine, with a mind filled with egoic concerns. In the second stage of meditation, we begin to move between sleep and wakefulness; here, the ego begins to loosen. As concentration is perfected, our "inner eye" gradually begins to open and we have spiritual experiences (here understood to be glimpses of the divine) that further loosen the hold of ego and awaken our true yearning for union. From this stage we move into "gnosis of the universe," a deepening of knowledge of reality and its many facets, which might include the development of intuitive and energetic powers. From here, the soul begins to experience stages associated with the "gnosis of the creator," subtler and subtler mystic experiences of the divine. Finally, a lucky few attain *fana fillah*, or "extinction of the self in Allah." While this is experienced within meditation, an even rarer few progress to *baqaa billah* and are

--- --- --- --- --- --- --- --- --- -- --

45. Franklin Lewis, "Rumi's Masnavi, Part 6: Unity of Being," *The Guardian*, January 4, 2010. https://www.theguardian.com/commentisfree/belief/2010/jan/04/rumi-masnavi-unity -being.

able to maintain this state while engaged in daily life, seeing in all that is a reflection of the divine face of Allah.

Practice

- - - - - - - - - -

DEVOTIONAL MEDITATION

Both St. Teresa and Rumi describe their spiritual experiences in terms of their "beloved." Devotion can be a powerful force in meditation. To experiment with this, try the following meditation:

- To begin, bring to mind a being for whom you feel immense love and affection (similar to the emotional chakra access method described in this chapter's first practice). This can be a spiritual being or deity if you have this feeling toward one, but also can simply be a loved one (human, animal, or other) in your life.

- Notice the feeling of this affection as an energy in your body (usually centered in the heart chakra, though you may feel it other places too).

- Particularly focus in on the feeling of *longing* connected to it—the desire to be with, or draw to you, your beloved.

- Once this feeling is strong, let go of the visual of the being you were focusing upon, and meditate on this feeling of longing itself, imagining it is now reaching for union with spirit itself.

- Sink into this feeling of longing for spirit (however you define it) and allow it to carry you wherever it will.

Contemplations

- Which model(s) of progression that we have covered in the last three chapters resonate the most with you?

- Have you experienced kundalini sensations in meditation (regardless of whether you practice kundalini meditation)? Do you relate to processing in terms of one or more of the chakras?

- Do you find symbolic representations of the spiritual progression, such as the esoteric reading of the *Egyptian Book of the Dead* presented here, helpful? What symbols are the most meaningful to you?

- What do you find of interest in Saint Teresa's mansions, or the Kabbalah Tree of Life, or the Sufi Maqamat?

- How has reading about traditions other than your own shifted your perceptions about your own meditation journey?

PART III
THE PATH

The path into the light seems dark,
the path forward seems to go back,
the direct path seems long
—*Tao Te Ching*[46]

We've all felt this way at times—about our meditation practice, our personal growth, or life. It's not always easy to see how meditation is helping us or that we are making any progress. Meditation may shine a spotlight on our awareness such that we won't like what we see. Sometimes the act of sitting down to quiet our mind allows space for long buried emotions or thought patterns to surface, and we are finally forced to deal with them. Other times we may just lose motivation and need help rediscovering or cultivating it again.

Part III focuses on these kinds of challenges—emotional disturbances, energetic sensitivity, recurring disturbing thoughts or images, and dry spells. Chapter 8 is about common traps or ruts we can fall into through meditation—siddhis and powers, attachment to attainment, spiritual bypassing and

---

46. Stephen Mitchel (translator), *Tao Te Ching,* (New York: Harper and Row, 1988), Aphorism 41.

disassociation, and intellectualization and conceptualization. Chapter 9 covers how retreat and pilgrimage may augment your path, and how to decide what is right for you if you feel you'd prefer more intensive practice in this form.

Meditation is so personal; it can be difficult to talk about some of these challenges because we're often advised not to judge our meditations. But without judgment and reevaluation, we can get stuck in a rut that could be avoided. You have to find the balance for yourself, between assessing your practice and letting go into whatever is happening for you. I offer this guide to some challenges and traps as a tool for asking yourself honest questions about your practice. But sometimes you just have to let go and trust your inner compass to take you where you need to be. Like so much of what has been covered, this too is a balance between navigation and surrender, effort and relaxation, discipline and trust.

SEVEN

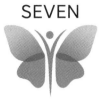

SUBTLER CHALLENGES

Nineteenth-century Indian yogi Paramahansa Ramakrishna said of meditation, "When a tree is young, it should be fenced all around; otherwise it may be destroyed by cattle."[47] He was exhorting his young students to engage in formal sitting meditation, not only the devotional and ritual practices they enjoyed so much. He explained to them that a daily meditation practice was a protected time each day when they could center "in the chamber of their hearts" without risk of getting "eaten up" by the world.[48]

Most of the time, meditation *does* feel like a protected space, a refuge from the stresses of daily life. But there are times it feels like the opposite—it heightens our sensitivity and the pain of being in the world intensifies instead of fading away. If we have come to meditation to relieve our suffering, be it physical, emotional, or spiritual, this increased sensitivity may be unwelcome or cause us to question the value of our practice. It is one of the many paradoxes of a regular meditation practice that it both strengthens our resilience and heightens our sensitivity to the world. It is essential to learn

- - - - - - - - - - - -

47. Swami Nikhilananda, *The Gospel of Sri Ramakrishna*, (New York: Ramakrishna-Vivekananda Center, 1942), 181.

48. Ibid.

to work with heightened sensitivity, be gentle with ourselves, and look into what may be going on within when it occurs.

In meditation, we strive to quiet our mind and detach from our everyday thoughts and concerns. As we practice this quiet for longer periods, we begin to notice patterns—thoughts we return to again and again, or the emotions underlying these thought patterns. What arises for us in meditation reflects and at times magnifies what is arising in the rest of our lives. If we are anxious about something, our mind will likely repeatedly return to it in meditation. Depending on the modality we are working with, we may simply pull our mind away from the anxious thought and go back to our object of meditation, or we may investigate that thought a bit—how does it feel in the body? Does it affect our breathing? In inquiry paths, we might even locate where in our mind or body this anxiety is arising from, and "who" is experiencing it. This line of inquiry works for many different emotional patterns and the thoughts they generate, whether it's anger, desire, fear, jealousy, or even hope and love.

Regardless of the form, through meditation we seek to change our relationship to these patterns, one thought at a time. In that process, there are many ways our psyche may react. We may resist change at some level, because even an emotional pattern that has caused us pain is familiar, and the unknown scarier by comparison. Or perhaps the emotional pattern we seek to release is self-protective and we fear on some level how letting go might affect us. We may become angry with ourselves or others, or fixate on blame (again, ourselves or others) for how the emotional pattern developed. We may become self-righteous and insistent that we are fully justified in feeling the way we do, regardless of whether it is of benefit to us. Or we may despair and believe our patterns are worse than everyone else's and are entirely unchangeable.

Should our resistance unfold on an unconscious level, it may play out in other ways. We may inwardly put the brakes on, wherein we halt our progress in meditation—maybe we convince ourselves that we are too busy to practice or just space out or think a lot while practicing day after day. We may begin to use meditation solely as a means of escape, wherein we repeatedly return to a particular state that feels pleasant, effectively stopping any real growth. We may grasp on to our meditation to bolster our ego and focus on creating or forcing mystic states as a sign of advancement, but this behavior is a form of self-medication (and really, avoidance) of the fears and insecurities we are feeling.

If we look at the process of shifting our conditioned patterns from the perspective of those traditions that acknowledge energy body teachings, we can see how other complications might arise. The energy body's different levels hold these patterns as obstructions or blocks, and as we strive to change, releases and reorganization happen at these levels. Some energy body levels hold karmic patterns; as the shifts we bring about touch these levels, they reverberate through our entire being. Our energy body functions as a link between our mind, body, and spirit, so any shifts on one level may reflect on another. We might experience emotional swings or physical symptoms as our energy body adjusts and realigns. A processing and integration phase needs to occur; as it does, we may experience side effects we find uncomfortable.

While these kinds of challenges are real, it's important not to seek them out or assume you must experience them. I remember one group meditation retreat I attended where many participants seemed to one-up each other in terms of the challenges they were facing, offered up as proof they were "going through something big" or "in the midst of a big release." I've seen people jump from one retreat or workshop to another in a constant search for the next catharsis. While releases and cathartic experiences certainly can be transformative, much of the growth from meditation happens in a much quieter—and joyful—way.

Identifying our levels of resistance is only half the path; as we make efforts to do so, challenges will naturally arise, wherein we usually need advice for dealing with them. Depending on what arises for you, you may need the help of a qualified therapist, guide, or teacher. I've already emphasized the particular importance of this kind of help if you have experienced trauma in your life. Complementary and post-meditation practices may also be of tremendous help—tools for integrating or diving deeper into patterns we can do on our own (some of these are covered in the final chapter). This chapter's focus is on some of the main ways our resistance to growth may manifest in our meditations—as increased emotional sensitivity, energetic sensitivity or disruptions, repetitive disturbing or intrusive thoughts, and dry spells or plateaus. You will also find pragmatic ways of dealing with each you can try.

Emotional Sensitivity

Emotional sensitivity may show up *in* our meditation—strong emotions within us related to some thought or experience had while meditating—or we may feel especially emotionally sensitive *after* our meditation, wherein we find ourselves easily triggered or overwhelmed by people in our lives or stimuli in our environment. Either way, strong emotions are a signal to pause and take stock of our situation.

If you experience a strong upwell of emotion in your meditation, it may need to be worked with differently from the manner in which you usually handle passing thoughts and emotions. Of course, in meditation of any form, when we catch ourselves in an internal dialogue or narrative, we let it go and examine or work with it as we've been instructed or return to our object of focus. But if overwhelming feelings of grief, sadness, anger, or fear arise, we may not be able to let go of it, and it may not be in our best interests to do so. These sorts of feelings may signal a need to work with the triggers for this emotion in a more in-depth way, including outside of meditation. So how do we know? How do we know when we should just try to let go of an emotion, let it move through us, or look at it more deeply?

To answer this question, let's first think about what may trigger a strong emotion based on what we have already covered in this book:

- **The surfacing of a long-buried memory.** As we learned in chapter 3, meditation can be a valuable component of trauma therapy because it helps us connect to our nonreactive mind and aids in our ability to work through trauma triggers. However, sometimes the very openness of meditation and the clearing away of mental clutter allows long-buried memories to rise from the depths of the mind, thereby triggering a strong reaction. We may experience a full memory or just a glimpse along with the strong emotion.

- **A repressed reaction to a recent event.** Similar to the arise of long-buried emotions, sometimes life is so busy that we do not process our emotions or emotional reactions to an event when it is occurring; it is only once we are able to slow down for our meditation practice that our true emotion is able to come forward. For example, we may suddenly realize we were very hurt by something our partner said to us the day before and find ourselves experiencing that hurt in our meditation, on something like tape delay.

- **The processing of a strong obstruction—a deeply conditioned pattern.** As covered in chapter 6, within energy-based traditions it is taught that karmas and conditioned emotional patterns are held in our energy body and that as meditation shifts the energetic vibrations and flows within us, it sometimes causes energy structures associated with these patterns to move and release. As this process occurs, we may experience an emotional reaction or catharsis as a side effect.

- **A magnified response to an internal narrative.** If we get caught up in a story in our head while meditating, our increased sensitivity and energy level may magnify our usual response. For example, if we are replaying an event from the day before that irritated us, we may find ourselves triggered into an even angrier state within meditation due to our heightened sensitivity, focus, and energy.

An important part of knowing how to handle a strong emotional uprising is assessing what is causing your reaction. It may be helpful to ask these three questions: (1) Is this recurring? (2) Does it feel cathartic? and (3) Does it trigger or is it accompanied by thoughts of overwhelm or self-harm? Depending on your answers, you can decide whether the emotion is something you want to work with outside of meditation through a healing or psychological modality, as well as whether you need additional support or help to do so. If a strong emotion recurs often in meditation, does not feel cathartic, and/or triggers or is accompanied by thoughts of overwhelm or self-harm, it's essential that you work with it outside of meditation through another means, and in the case of self-harm, seek professional support right away.

As we've already discussed, a regular meditation practice is a part of our overall emotional growth and healing trajectory, and often we will find that complementary modalities are helpful. This might be healing modalities such as body work or energy work, psychological modalities such as talk therapy or group counseling, or combination modalities that involve somatic processing of emotions in the body. When you are going through a phase of experiencing strong emotions in your meditation, it is often a sign that you need to pursue other ways of working with these emotions in your body, psyche, and subtle body. The right modality for you is individual to you, based on your proclivities and preferences as well as whatever is causing the emotion. If you are not sure what modality might be helpful to you, consider the resources in the book list for ideas.

No matter how you proceed, it is important is to be gentle and understanding with yourself, both within your meditation and outside of it. Because of the emphasis on nonattachment in meditation training, there is a tendency to feel that we should dismiss all emotions, no matter how strongly they arise, and that we have somehow "failed" if we cannot do so. Tamping down your emotions is never helpful and may even cause them to magnify or express in the form of physical illness or stresses down the road. If an emotion within your meditation becomes overwhelming, don't feel you need to sit through it! Allow yourself to get up from your cushion and engage in activities you find soothing. Talk to a friend, read a favorite book, take a bath—do what feels right.

Sometimes when experiencing catharsis, all we need to do is sit and let ourselves have a good cry. You will know if you are experiencing a release in this way; despite the emotional intensity, it feels as if it is *moving through*. There are other times we need to reach out for support and comfort right away, and work with the root of the emotion at a later time. Remember that you are engaged in a process of self-discovery, not self-conquest. And as covered in the section on trauma-sensitivity within chapter 3, if you have any history of trauma, you want to be especially gentle and kind with yourself.

Another kind of emotional sensitivity that can arise happens after emerging from a meditation. I have experienced mornings where after a perfectly peaceful meditation session, I walk into my kitchen and find myself snapping at my husband or kids. What is going on when this occurs? Sometimes the very openness and peace we touch in meditation makes the "normal" stimuli of our everyday lives seem abrasive. If we are at all attached to the feelings experienced in our meditation—that is, if we grip them and try to hold on to them—we will react with rigidity or irritation as soon as we encounter any other feeling or energies. These moments are a message to us that show us where we are holding, and where we can let go more. The point is to carry our meditation-found peace and insight into our interactions and daily activities.

Allowing ourselves transition time, if possible, can be the key to minimizing this kind of post-meditation triggering. Create a transition ritual, such as a few light stretches or even brushing your teeth between the end of your meditation and before you engage with others. This transition ritual can be almost anything, as long as it is the same after every meditation session. Much like the pre-meditation ritual (covered in chapter 2), if you repeat it every day it will signal to your psyche and mind that you are shifting into another gear. It will also allow your energy body to re-anchor in preparation for interaction with others.

The whole point of meditation is the integration of what you experience into the way you meet the world. Our whole life is our meditation practice, and we are training for handling triggers and emotions every time we sit down. We have not failed when we become triggered; these moments are learning opportunities. As with emotions that arise during your meditation, it's important to be gentle and inquisitive with yourself. Look into the causes, and don't berate yourself. We are like that young tree Ramakrishna spoke of, entering a protected space each day during our meditation. And when we get up from our cushion, we ultimately take the fence down and engage directly with the world. We do the best we can to meet that world with openness, tranquility, and wisdom, learning as we go.

Practice

- - - - - - - - - - -

ASSESSING EMOTIONAL INTENSITY

- If you experience emotional intensity during your meditation, take a break, treat yourself with gentle self-care, and assess.
- If the experience is a recurring one, feels overwhelming, or triggers a desire to self-harm, seek support.

- If it feels cathartic, it may be a byproduct of a energetic and/or karmic release—allow it to move through, and treat yourself with sensitivity afterwards.

- At a later point, get curious with yourself about what the roots of this emotional release are, using the list in this section (memory, recent situation, delayed response, and so on).

- If you often feel emotionally sensitive after your meditation, create a post-meditation ritual to help your transition.

Energy Bursts and Sensitivity

The energy or subtle body serves as an intermediary between the mind and physical body. Regardless of whether or not we engage in energy-based meditation forms such as kundalini and chakra practices, shifts in our subtle body naturally occur over time as we meditate. Most of the time these shifts are gradual; we may not even feel them. Usually when we do feel them, it is as pleasant sensations of warmth, contentment, or even bliss. But once in a while we may experience energy bursts, within or outside of meditation, that feel jarring. This is different from the kundalini crises mentioned in chapter 6 because there are no serious physical or mental problems that accompany them. Usually these energy bursts occur for a period of days but can be longer; as energy flows through our subtle body in a new way, blockages are dissolved, and we adjust to the new configuration. Some common symptoms of this kind of adjustment, all of which may occur while meditating or outside of it, are:

- Spontaneous jerking or twitching of a body part or your whole body, similar to when you jerk or start awake after dozing off but haven't been asleep.

- A feeling of pressure or intensity in one or more chakras, or in any other part of your body. This is not physical pain, but instead feels distinctly like an energy.

- A rush or surge of energy somewhere in your body, sometimes accompanied by a shortening of breath or muscle contraction.

- A sensation that your body is growing larger or lighter, and/or that you may burst out of your skin.

- Intense heat rising up your torso, engulfing your head, or anywhere else in your body.

- Spontaneous sexual arousal, when no sexual stimulant (mental or physical) is present.

While these experiences may be unusual, they shouldn't alarm you. They are part of the natural process of your mind and body transforming. In a way, we are going through a kind of upgrade process, and our system needs to adjust to the new software. Reminding yourself of this will help you relax, and often this relaxation in and of itself will also cause the energy bursts to stabilize or lessen. The emotion of alarm creates a tension that heightens the discomfort.

If within your meditation you find you are really uncomfortable with whatever is occurring, here are a few things to try:

- **Change things up.** If you meditate with closed eyes, open them and look around for a few seconds or minutes. If you meditate with open eyes, close them and visualize a soothing place.

- **Move.** Sway back and forth, stretch, or even stand up and walk around to see if this will help to dissipate the sensation.

- **Shift your meditation anchor.** If you use a mantra, change to a visual; if you are using a visual, change to a mantra. If you focus on your breath, chant a mantra or use a visual for a while. Even a few deep, long chants of *om* can help.

- **Take a few very deep breaths,** lifting your arms high above your body as you do so and tensing your muscles, relaxing everything at once while you drop your arms. Repeat as often as you like.

- **Stop.** If you are very uncomfortable, end your meditation and do something else. As always, don't judge and don't self-blame. Just let it be.

If your energy bursts are recurring over a period of time, there are things you can do outside of meditation to help to stabilize your energy body and speed your adjustment time:

- **Move more.** Increase your exercise routine, and/or go for regular walks. This will get the energy moving through your physical.
- **Try yoga or tai chi.** Now is a great time to give these mind-body modalities a try, if you haven't already. They are designed to smooth and purify the energy currents of the body.
- **Water.** Drink more, bathe more, swim more. Even sitting by large bodies of water will help. Water has a cleansing, balancing energy that is particularly helpful for this kind of energetic processing (of course drink water in healthy, not overwhelming, amounts).
- **Hang out with a tree.** Really any time in nature will help, but trees in particular have a balancing and stabilizing quality.
- **Increase your protein intake.** Protein is naturally grounding and smooths our vibrational frequency. Of course, do not artificially inflate your protein levels above what is healthy. Just increase it a bit if there is healthy room to do so within your diet.
- **Ground energetically.** Try the practice that follows, or something similar.

If any of the symptoms persist for long or they become overly bothersome, consider consulting a body worker, energy worker, spiritual guide, or therapist for help in diagnosing and processing what is occurring. And no matter what you do, remember that these bursts are generally a sign of changes and shifts—a spiritual growing pain, if you will.

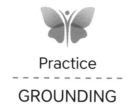

Practice

GROUNDING

The following grounding visualization can be helpful when experiencing a buildup of energy intensity in your meditation:

- Notice where in your body you are most feeling the intensity. Identify its shape and size and even color if it feels relevant.
- On your exhales, imagine this energy is gradually leaving your body through your base, into the earth. You can stand for this if you like and imagine it is leaving through your feet, or if you remain seated, see it leaving through your tailbone and legs.
- Now imagine the earth is emanating up a soothing, calming, stabilizing energy—first into your feet, legs, and tailbone and then into your entire body. You feel calmer and your energy feels smoother as you do so.
- Return to your core meditation if you like.

Disturbing Thoughts or Images

Occasionally you may experience disturbing or unwanted thoughts or images in your meditation, sometimes recurring for a period of time, similar to recurring nightmares. These are what psychologists call "intrusive thoughts"—spontaneous thoughts that distress us in some way. These may be thoughts of harming yourself or others, or thoughts that you consider sexually or religiously inappropriate. If you have these kinds of intrusive thoughts regularly and they disturb you, it can be a sign of an obsessive-compulsive disorder that requires professional help. Much of the time, however, intrusive thoughts are not indicative of anything; they are simply the mind generating activity. Psychological research shows that everyone experiences some intrusive thoughts and they are rarely linked to deep-seated issues. In fact, it is often our reaction to an intrusive thought that determines whether or not it will recur: if we are alarmed by it or it generates an emotional reaction, a "hook" is created and the thought is more likely to recur.

How do you know whether you are simply experiencing an intrusive thought or some larger emotional work needs to be done? An intrusive thought initially seems random and does not have an emotional intention or charge behind it. We may *react* to the thought emotionally, but when it first arises it is surprising and usually does not seem tied to anything going on in our life. For example, if you suddenly have an image of punching your neighbor but haven't actually felt any anger toward him or have any reason to do so, then there's no emotional charge or intention to it. It's just a thought your mind has randomly generated. However, if you become alarmed by this thought, feel instant guilt, judge yourself as a "terrible person," or start searching for why you may unconsciously be harboring hatred for your neighbor, you have now fed that thought, and it is much more likely to happen again.

On the other hand, if you have had a recent argument with your neighbor and thoughts of punching him have the emotional feeling of anger behind them—there's a charge. The thought or image is an *expression* of your anger or irritation. In this case, maybe you do need to work with your anger a little bit. Maybe you need to work with it in your body, right there in your meditation, or talk it through with someone afterwards. Maybe you need to physically discharge your anger through exercise.

If a thought is truly an "uncharged" thought rather than an intrusive one, the key to working with it is the same as with all the other more mundane thoughts that arise—don't touch it. This is exactly what therapists working with clients with intrusive thought disorders teach their patients to do; in other words, these patients learn a form of meditation, or at least a meditative relationship to their thoughts in the moment. When you refrain from feeding a thought attention, it will naturally subside. Don't treat a violent or sexual or politically incorrect thought any differently than a thought about what you are going to have for dinner or what you are going to wear to work. Just let it be.

As for why the mind generates these kinds of thoughts, we do not really know. In meditation, it can sometimes feel like your own mind is trying to test you. Rachel is a friend who has meditated for more than thirty years, and is a very wonderful, warm, and open practitioner. Recently, however, she told me she was disturbed by a recurring series of images of herself eating meat. She is a devout vegan and has been for almost as long as she has meditated. At times, she has had to work with releasing her judgment and anger at those who work in the meat industry, eat meat, or harm animals. She has let go of this anger and has instead learned to use her anger in a compassionate and nonjudgmental way (she is very active in the animal rights community). But in meditation, her mind suddenly started generating all these images of herself eating meat, which she found extremely disturbing. She began to wonder what it meant and felt guilty just for having these thoughts.

Did she secretly want meat? Was it symbolic of some other harmful intention within her? Was she punishing herself with these thoughts? For many of us, thoughts of eating meat would not be the most disturbing thing our mind could throw at us. But for her it was…and that is exactly the point. The mind sometimes presents to us exactly whatever is the hardest for us to *not touch*.

In these cases, the best approach is to stay calm and breathe—this is not a prescription to push or will yourself through the thought. At the same time, don't overanalyze unless you really believe there is an emotional intention or charge behind your disturbing thought or image that warrants more inquiry. In Rachel's case, the breakthrough came when she stopped inquiring and was able to laugh at herself. One day she was sitting in meditation when the image of herself eating meat arose and she just found it funny. She suddenly realized just how much time she had spent obsessing over this thought, analyzing it and questioning it, and really it was just another wave in her mind. The trickery of this cracked her up. We really are very funny creatures, and meditation will prove that to you over and over again!

This light-hearted ending is obviously not intended to dismiss more serious obsessive-compulsive disorders that some people experience or the arising of long-buried traumatic memories as covered earlier in this chapter. If your disturbing thoughts recur and you are not able to work through them, of course you should seek support and help. Have the honesty and courage to recognize when you need help.

Practice

WORKING WITH DISTURBING THOUGHTS

- If you find yourself experiencing a strong disturbing thought or image in meditation, try not to give it additional fuel through your reaction.

- Separate the image or thought from your reaction to the image or thought. If you need to stop meditating to do this, then do so.

- Assess whether or not the thought/image has an emotional charge, and/ or whether or not it is linked to an actual event or feeling you have. Then decide how to work with it accordingly.

- If you experience recurring thoughts/images that do not seem linked to any event or feeling, try to relax into them. Switch up your meditation form if needed (change your anchor for example) for a few days to break the momentum.

Dry Spells

Perhaps you have read through this chapter so far and thought, "I *wish* I was experiencing some of these challenges…at least then I'd know something is happening in my meditation! Right now, it's just a slog, day after day, always the same; nothing new or exciting ever happens. I'm not even sure it's doing me any good at all…maybe I should just sleep in." Yep, we've all been there. A dedicated meditation practice is a lot like a cross-country drive—occasionally you hit a particularly scenic or congested patch of road, but mostly it's just a whole lot of flat, empty landscape. It's interesting that many of the maps for the spiritual journey we examined in the last chapter incorporate a metaphor for this phase—"waiting in line" within the *Egyptian Book of Coming Forth by Day,* Saint Teresa's Third Mansion, and the daily work of the yamas in Patanjali's path.

I find that of all the questions that arise regarding meditation, the question of what to do when you are feeling unmotivated is the one that generates the most disagreement. Some teachers will say to take a break and wait until you miss meditating to return. The logic behind this is that forcing ourselves to meditate only generates more internal resistance that could eventually intensify and turn into some form of self-sabotage. You may grow to resent your meditation practice so much that it becomes impossible to return to. If you take a break, this line of thinking goes, eventually some part of you will pull you back to practice when the time is right.

Other teachers and traditions instruct basically to just power through— use your willpower and maintain your meditation routine. If you give up the routine, it's all too easy for it to slip away entirely, and then even once you want to return, you may find yourself unable to get in the habit again. With regularity and commitment, this line of thinking goes, you will naturally pass through the phase of lack of motivation. Something will happen in your life that reignites your meditation, you will turn to it as a true refuge once again, or something new will naturally arise.

For myself and many people I have worked with, I find a compromise is often best—keep the routine but allow yourself to take a break from whatever form you have been engaging in to try a different one. I believe it is important to keep a meditation routine. I have seen too many people take a break and regret it when they confront the difficulty of establishing the routine again once they desire to start again. On the other hand, I also believe that sometimes we need to shake things up. In some traditions, this stance of compromise is more controversial than you might imagine, and it is true that it is generally unhelpful to approach meditation as a sampler might, e.g., trying chakra meditation for a few months, then insight meditation for a bit, then mantra. Meditation forms unfold over time, and it is best to stick with one form for long enough to plumb its depths.

If you are truly feeling unmotivated, allow yourself a break from your current form, and experiment. Even the process of researching other forms is often enough to reignite motivation. There is such a richness of meditations available to us nowadays, and so many guided forms available. Usually engaging in a new form for a few weeks or months will break a dry spell and returning to your core practice will feel like returning home. Sometimes, experimenting may lead you in a new direction entirely, wherein you will realize that it's time for a new core practice.

Personally, I've had two core practices over the course of my thirty-plus years of meditating: first a chakra- and kundalini-based practice for twenty years, and in the last decade Tibetan Buddhist practices. Over these decades I have also studied and practiced other forms, most notably mindfulness, insight, and *tonglen* (a Tibetan compassion practice) for weeks or months at a time. I have always found shifting to a new practice for a period of time to be re-motivating and transformative, and doing so helped me discover attachments to my core practices or ways I was holding or seeking the creation of experiences rather than allowing them to happen. Sometimes you can only see ways you are using your meditation as a crutch, or ways you are attached to experiences you are having once you have let go. Experimenting with a new form of meditation for a time is a way to maintain your routine while creating an opportunity to refresh and revitalize your practice. When you return to your original method, it will be fresh and informed by your new perspective.

For those for whom meditation has become a lifelong practice, it's normal to experience one or more core shifts. If we hold too tightly to one core practice, we may miss the chance for a fruitful change. A useful tool for assessing whether you are in need of a bigger change is to ask yourself what your current motivation for meditating is and whether it has changed. If you came to meditation for medical reasons and it has now become part of a spiritual quest, is your spirit being fed, or do you need more? If you were searching for answers and meaning through meditation, are you now feeling disillusioned for some reason, and do you need to approach it from a new angle? What is going on in your life and what do you need right now? Being honest about these questions will help you get to the deeper issues under your current dry spell, and may help you determine how to handle it.

While a permanent change is sometimes necessary, in most cases taking a break from your core practice to experiment with others will be transitory. Taking this approach will allow you to maintain the power of your meditation routine while generating some new enthusiasm to practice. And enthusiasm *is* necessary—maybe not every day but definitely overall. We are often told not to focus on outcome in meditation, and certainly this is good advice. I am also a firm believer that a natural byproduct of meditation is enjoyment— itself a natural state of being. However fleeting those feelings of wholeness, tranquility, relaxation, and/or bliss may be, they are glimpses into our true nature, something our being craves. While we will cover the problems with becoming *attached* to these states in the next chapter, they are still a part of the meditation journey; if they are completely absent for you, reevaluate what you are doing and find a form that brings some enjoyment back. An increase in self-awareness and kindness off the cushion is just as much a reflection of our natural state, so if you are not experiencing these, again it may be time to reevaluate. Allow yourself this gift—for meditation *is* a gift you give yourself.

Contemplations

• Think back over your history with meditation. Have you experienced phases of resistance? How did they resolve?

• Have you ever experienced heightened emotions during meditation, or soon after? Looking back did it seem to be caused by any of the examples given here? How did you work through it? Which of the suggestions offered here would you like to try in the future?

• Have you ever experienced energy bursts or heightened energy sensitivity during meditation or during a phase of your life since beginning meditating? What do you now see as happening, and how did it resolve? Which of the suggestions offered here would you like to try in the future?

• Have you had, or are you experiencing, a "dry spell" in your meditation? Do you feel you need to re-examine your motivations and experiment with a new form? What has helped you in the past, or what might help you now?

• Are you connected to the natural enjoyment of meditation most of the time? If not, what can you do to reconnect with this joy?

EIGHT

MYSTIC STATES AND COMMON MEDITATION TRAPS

Spiritual seekers throughout history have described profound and at times dramatic mystic states experienced in meditation. Many were covered in part II—yogic samadhis, Buddhist jhanas, kundalini blisses, St. Teresa's "prayer of quiet," and Sufi divine union. You might experience mystic states outside of formal religious practice as well, and as we've seen from the research of neuroscientist Dr. Andrew Newberg explored in chapter 3, the human brain actually seems hardwired for them. But what exactly *are* mystic experiences?

Late nineteenth-/early twentieth-century philosopher and psychologist William James, perhaps the first to attempt to categorize such experiences across multiple spiritual traditions, noted that all have two primary features: they are *ineffable*, unobtainable through the intellect and indescribable; and they are *noetic*, containing knowledge, importance, and wisdom that to the experiencer feels revelatory and cannot be known any other way. He identifies two additional frequent features of mystic experience: it is *transient*, a state one emerges from; and people feel *passive* within it, i.e., the sense that something is being *received* or a feeling of being swept up into the experience, not creating it through any effort.[49] These features as a definition of mystic experience hold up remarkably well when assessing spiritual states of all kinds, and they aid us in asking the most pertinent questions as meditators: What is the meaning of such experiences? What is their value, and the proper relationship to them? Should we seek or avoid them in meditation?

The answer depends on who you ask, how long you have been meditating (in some cases), where you are on your path, and the nature of the experience. For example, mindfulness meditation practitioners are often initially instructed to let go of such experiences and consider them as just another mental phenomenon arising, best left untouched. Yet as we saw in chapter 5 on the jhanas, even within traditions that practice mindfulness there is a place for this kind of mystic experience and for active training in its cultivation. Remember that the jhanas are not considered end states in and of themselves; they are preparatory—helpful in developing the concentration necessary to obtain true wisdom through insight practice and purifying as they loosen the holds of the conditioned mind that block realization. What jhanic teachings are very emphatic about is something William James also noted about them—they are *transient* and therefore not the final goal. Mystic states are a means to an end, a tool to aid us along the way.

In fact, the same could be said of all the paths we've covered; all contain descriptions of multiple mystic states one might experience on the spiritual journey *but* the final stage is one in which these experiences no longer come and go. The realizations obtained through them become a permanent way of being. In the yogic path, the samadhis all the way up through nibija/nirivkalpa samadhi (complete dissolution of self) are still transient—a meditator emerges from the experience. Only in the final stage, sahaja samadhi, does this "in and out" feeling cease, becoming a natural way of being rather than a transient state. The field of reeds in the *Egyptian Book of Coming Forth by Day,* da'at in Kabbalah, the seventh mansion in St. Teresa's system, and baqaa billah in Sufism—these final stages in all of these maps represent a movement beyond the transitory nature of the mystic experiences that precede them.

----

49. William James, *Varieties of Religious Experience,* (New York: Cosimo Classics, 2004), 109. Originally published 1902 by Longmans, Greens & Co.

From a spiritual perspective then, this provides us important insight into how to relate to mystic experiences, regardless of our tradition: Don't be fooled into stopping at a certain state and simply returning to it over and over, no matter how wonderful it is—it is not the end. Don't become attached. This is part of the purpose of progressive guided paths, the kinds of maps of the spiritual journey covered in part II, as well as the role of a good teacher (explored in chapter 10)—they help us realize there is more, and we shouldn't settle or get stuck. The ability to move in and out of these states at will is often cultivated in formal yogic and jhanic programs as a means of strengthening the mind but also as a means of ensuring attachments don't form and these states can be released. Understanding this is important for deepening our practice.

But what if your motivation in meditation is not spiritual? What if you are meditating for health or stress management purposes and are not really interested in the highest states as defined by the world's religious traditions? Is there value in learning to enter and stay in one state day after day in your meditation? The answer is more complicated. As covered in chapter 3, research does show that once we have obtained a certain level of concentration, most object-based meditation forms induce the relaxation response in our body: our breathing slows, our muscles relax, production of stress hormones declines, and production of endorphins may increase. Relaxing in this way is profoundly good for us and doing it daily even more so. It can lower our average stress "set point"—the average level of the stress hormones in our system on a daily basis—which, in turn, lowers our susceptibility to stress-based health problems. In this sense, seeking out this state and learning to return to it daily does have benefits. And although this state is perhaps not exactly mystic, realizing its benefits demonstrates how much motivation influences the answer to the question of how to handle meditation states and experiences.

However, the answer is different if we are practicing another form that can help greatly with stress management: mindfulness. Generally when practicing mindfulness, we don't seek to cultivate any particular state or experience or to hold on to one that arises. This aids us in stress management in another way—it is practice for noticing and not attaching ourselves to emotions that stressful situations may trigger. You may recall from chapter 3 that this noticing of emotions allows us to choose a response rather than react from a conditioned mind. In this form, letting go of mystic experience is another sort of training in letting go of distraction, staying present in the here and now, and learning to navigate our daily lives with the same level of present awareness.

On the other hand, it's taught within many energy healing traditions that entering into certain vibrational fields (whether through chakra meditation or visualizations) and staying there to absorb healing energies can have a profound and powerful healing effect. And within kundalini-based traditions, spending certain amounts of time in various states of bliss is considered cathartic and purifying, such that the resulting bliss is a natural byproduct of obstructions releasing. This point of view is found in teachings on both the jhanas and the samadhis as well. So, as to whether we should seek these states or not and how we should relate to them, it once again depends very much on your motivation and where you are in your path. Mystic states have value—not the least of which is enjoyment that can greatly increase a motivation to meditate—but they also can become traps in which we become stuck. Indeed, most of the remainder of this chapter explores the many ways we can get stuck by mystic experience: attachment to attainment, spiritual bypassing, and disassociation, to name a few.

But before we get into that topic, let's explore another feature of mystic experience as William James defined it—what he called its noetic quality or its ability to impart wisdom. Beyond simple purification or motivation, within many traditions mystic experience is seen to convey knowledge unknowable in any other way. Through meditation we gradually let go of our usual way of knowing—through words, thoughts, and the conditioned mind—and open to other modes. Trappist monk Thomas Merton put it beautifully (he uses the phrase "contemplation" to refer to Christian forms of meditation):

> ...[C]ontemplation is a kind of spiritual vision to which both reason and faith aspire, by their very nature, because without it they must always remain incomplete. Yet con-

templation is not vision because it sees "without seeing" and knows "without knowing." It is a more profound depth of faith, a knowledge too deep to be grasped in images, in words, or even in clear concepts. It can be suggested by words, by symbols, but in the very moment of trying to indicate what it knows the contemplative mind takes back what it has said, and denies what it has affirmed. For in contemplation we know by "unknowing." Or, better, we know beyond all knowing or "unknowing."[50]

The manner in which we integrate what we come to know into our everyday mind is very individual and dependent upon tradition. To one person, the sense of being a passive receiver of the experience—another feature William James noted is often present in mystic experience—may be confirmation of a higher power, proof there is a divine bestower of grace. To another, that same passive/receptive quality may be experienced as a deep relaxation, a release of obstructions to enlightened mind. The common experience through all is of wisdom being gained, a veil being lifted, or realization arising. This wisdom transcends the actual experience; it is not just about pleasure, dramatic visions, energy rushes, or peaceful states. We feel we have understood something new. This kind of experience is valued by virtually every tradition and offers another important way we can assess how to relate to experiences we have: If they impart wisdom, they have value.

Practice

- - - - - - - - - - -

ASSESSING MYSTIC EXPERIENCE

When considering how to relate to any mystic or unusual experience that arises for you in meditation, ask yourself:

- - - - - - - - - - - -

50. Thomas Merton and Sue Monk Kidd, *New Seeds of Contemplation,* (New York: New Directions, 2007), 1–2.

- What is my motivation, and does this experience serve it?

- Am I attached to the search for and recreation of this experience's plea-sure for its own sake, which would therefore potentially keep me stuck? (A question covered in more depth in a later section.)

- Does it feel cathartic, purifying, or healing?

- Does it convey some wisdom or knowing that stays with me beyond my actual feelings while in meditation?

Siddhis and Powers

Siddhi is a Sanskrit word referring to paranormal or spiritual abilities that can arise through meditation. Patanjali details some of these himself in his *Yoga Sutras*, including clairvoyance, telepathy, recall of past lives, and even invisibility. Other common powers attributed to siddha masters in various yogic and Buddhist texts include levitation, astral travel, prophecy, telekine-sis, dream travel, healing, and the manifestation of magical substances such as sacred ash or nectar. While Patanjali and other teachers note that siddhis might be obtained through other means such as herbs or past life recall, they are primarily considered to be obtainable through intense training in certain forms of meditation. They might also arise spontaneously as a kind of side effect of a meditation practice.

Such powers are considered both natural *and* risky. Like mystic experi-ences, the siddhi are considered very tangible and organic extension of our consciousness—they involve working with levels of consciousness most of us are not aware of but are latent within everyone. And like mystic experi-ences, focusing on attaining siddhis can be at best a distraction and at worst dangerous. Both Hinduism and Buddhism teach that attachment to them can stunt spiritual growth, and, even worse, misuse of them can cause us to generate negative karmas that set us back further, possibly for lifetimes.

Other spiritual traditions have a similarly divided stance on such abilities. Within Christianity they have often been considered demonic, and many people were put to death as part of the Crusades after being accused of pos-sessing such powers. On the other hand, to be canonized as a Catholic saint an individual must have performed some miraculous act, and of course in the New Testament Jesus performs many. In these cases, such powers are considered displays of God's power—gifts coming through an individual, as opposed to powers they *possess*. Similar teachings exist in Kabbalah and Sufism as well. The general stance on siddhis or occult powers is similar— if they are sought for their own sake, used for harm, or attached to with pride, they are a serious spiritual obstacle. If they are used in service to others, including helping to affirm others' faith without attachment or pride, they are in spiritual alignment and possibly even miraculous. Telling the difference is not always so easy, and has often succumbed to larger historical forces, as evidenced by stories such as that of Joan of Arc, who was burnt at the stake by the Church for her mystic visions and then posthumously canonized as a saint with those same visions acknowledged as miraculous.

These days, there are many training programs out there to help individuals develop their intuition, healing abilities, dreaming capacity, and other skills that would be considered siddhis under the classic definition. Most include some kind of meditation practice but are not necessarily taught within a spiritual context. In one sense, developing these abilities is no different than developing any other skill that might be considered powerful in the world—an advanced degree in some topic, the ability to lead, or a high level of artistic or sports skill. These can all be used with either intent good or bad and for yourself or others—again, it all comes down to motivation. The risk of siddhis is that they function on a level other people do not necessarily see, and therefore the risk of misuse is greater, e.g., violating others' energetic boundaries without consent, or influencing events without realizing the full consequences. An ethical framework for working with these abilities and a profound self-awareness of our own capacity are both essential and should be the cornerstone of any training program for their cultivation.

From a meditation perspective, the danger mostly lies in us becoming attached to such abilities or mistaking them for a sign of spiritual advancement. In his famous *Autobiography of a Yogi*, Swami Yogananda tells us of meetings with many saints with miraculous abilities and warns us that such abilities are little more than parlor tricks. After describing his meeting with one yogi who could manifest scents he notes:

> [p]erformances of miracles such as shown by the "Perfume Saint" are spectacular but spiritually useless. Having little

purpose beyond entertainment, they are digressions from a
serious search for God.[51]

Of course, manifesting scents is not a siddhi most of us find spontaneously arising in our meditation or one we seek. For the average meditator,
siddhi development may be much more subtle, which is where the problem
lies, because we don't notice and therefore monitor our usage of our new
abilities. One of the most common ability is increased intuition, whether
psychic or simply based in the keener observatory abilities that come with
more present awareness, it's common to become much more attuned to what
others are feeling and even thinking through meditation. This attunement
can engender compassion as we gain a deeper understanding of what others
are going through, but it's also possible to begin subtly using this ability to
manipulate others or for personal gain, perhaps even unconsciously.

Preventing this requires a deep commitment to self-monitoring and
vigilance. As our meditation practice deepens, we should be developing a
corresponding increased awareness of the mind's daily activity outside of
meditation. If we are simply going into meditative states and then returning
to the same old conditioned mind, we will be prone to this kind of unconscious use of any new abilities that may arise wherein they will be co-opted
by our ego. Our awareness in meditation should be increasing our awareness of previously unconscious levels of intent, so we need to be observant of
these outside meditation as well. Within the context of what we've covered
in this book, this idea is nothing new; all the spiritual paths covered include
morality and ethics practices within which it is clear that attention to these
continues throughout the journey, not only in the initial stages. In fact, it's
often that the longer we meditate, the more essential these practices become
as they help prevent the slip into arrogance or the feeling of being beyond
or above morality. Ethics are a grounding and centering base from which
we can integrate any siddhis that arise or mystic experiences we have. As
discussed in the last chapter, it's common for obstacles or ego traps that arise

- - - - - - - - - - -

51. Paramahansa Yogananda, *Autobiography of a Yogi*, (Los Angeles: Self-Realization Fellow-
    ship, 2014), 45.

to require psychological or emotional work outside of meditation to help us truly uproot these tendencies.

The bottom line is that a meditation practice should increase our self-awareness and compassion. Though they may be disheartening to discover, we should understand our emotional triggers and patterns more clearly as we become more honest with ourselves about the moments of selfishness, arrogance, fear, or anger that underlies some of what we think and do. If we are working through these, our daily life and meditation practice fuel each other. As we practice noticing and letting go of subtler levels of mind and emotional patterns in our meditation, we become more aware of them as they arise in our daily lives and don't act them out. If we are doing this work, we are assured we won't misuse siddhis as they arise, as we are purifying our intent as we go. In essence, this is the whole path of personal growth through meditation, regardless of whether we are engaged in it within a spiritual tradition. And yes, sometimes it's trickier than you might imagine, so let's turn now to some of the ways we can trick ourselves.

Attachment to Attainment

As we covered in chapter 3, our brain is hardwired to respond to reward. The biological, brain-based tendency to respond to reward, desire the reward again, and come to anticipate and even seek it through repeating whatever behavior seemed to have brought it to us in the first place serves as the foundation for much of our conditioning. It is also the manner in which we can become stuck in meditation—that is, by becoming attached to and seeking to replicate a particular meditation state we find pleasant or satisfying. What kinds of states do we find satisfying or pleasant? This is very individual; for some it will be blissful states that release endorphins or rushes of pleasurable energy throughout our body. For others who perhaps find the world's stimuli overwhelming, experiences of a "void" or nothingness may be the most rewarding, as these feel like a relief from the bombardment of daily life. And still others who may feel trapped by their bodies or lives will find great relief in the feelings of boundarylessness. The point is, most of us will have some meditative state experienced as a "reward"; because it feels good to us, we will become attached and seek to replicate that feeling again and again.

The way in which this particular sort of longing keeps us stuck on our spiritual journey has been covered already, but it is mentioned here again because it is really only one of many ways that the reward-seeking cycle may trick us. Most of us are conditioned to want to succeed; most schooling is generally based on scores and grades. We compete in sports and other activities in which winning and being the best are what gets us acknowledgment. We might have other ways we seek the feeling of accomplishment—perhaps it's praise for our appearance, humor, or artistic abilities—for some it's even being bad or the worst. Whatever it is, we crave acknowledgment for it, that we are "good at it," a reward we are trapped in seeking. It is all too easy for us to relate to our meditation in the same way—we begin seeking this inner reward of feeling like we are moving forward, getting somewhere, attaining something. This feeling might manifest as pride in the amount we meditate or how disciplined we are, in the experiences we are having, a particular state we can access regularly, or even in how compassionate we are becoming.

Chögyam Trungpa, one of the first Tibetan Buddhist teachers in the West and founder of both Shambhala Training and Naropa University, coined the term "spiritual materialism" for this and related traps:

> Walking the spiritual path properly is a very subtle process; it is not something to jump into naively. There are numerous sidetracks which lead to a distorted, ego-centered version of spirituality; we can deceive ourselves into thinking we are developing spiritually when instead we are strengthening our egocentricity through spiritual techniques. This fundamental distortion may be referred to as spiritual materialism.[52]

As he notes, the main danger is believing that we are moving forward spiritually when actually we are moving backward. We think we are becoming less egoic but are really using our meditation to shore up our ego. What's actually happened is that we've just transferred our sense of identity and validation from worldly accomplishment to the spiritual path. Because meditations are a private affair, it's hard for anyone to call us on this identification

---

52. Chögyam Trungpa, *Cutting Through Spiritual Materialism,* (Boston: Shambhala, 2010), back cover.

or dispute our accomplishment. It's possible to live indefinitely in a world of our own making in which we are always progressing.

Seeing and releasing this identification is subtle, as is working with all these advanced meditation challenges. We first need to notice and honestly acknowledge the attachments we have. We can inquire into this ourselves by noticing whether or not there is a sense of reaching or striving for a particular state when we are meditating. Unless we are training in a system like the jhanas where we seek to consciously shift ourselves into particular states at will, or engage in a form of meditation in which we must construct a visualization, our meditation should never have this reaching or forced quality; these feelings are mind activity we are generating. We also need to look for and acknowledge thoughts and feelings of pride in relation to our practice and experiences. Momentary flashes of this are not a problem; as with everything that arises, it's our *attachment* to and subsequent reinforcement of these feelings when they arise that can become obstructive.

One of the best indicators of attachment to spiritual attainment is our feelings toward others and how they evolve. Are we becoming less judgmental and more understanding? Or are we developing an internal attitude of superiority and separateness that actually generates more judgment and less compassion? While seemingly simplistic, honestly answering these questions for ourselves can help reveal a lot of delusion in relation to our meditation. When we find signs of this attachment, the key is not to dramatically swing to the other end of the spectrum, into self-flagellation and self-denigration. These behaviors are the dark twin of arrogance and serve us no better than arrogance and judgment.

The antidote to feelings of superiority, arrogance, or spiritual attachment we find arising in ourselves is shifting our meditation practice to directly *counter* them. Practice compassion meditation for a time if you are finding yourself becoming judgmental, or equanimity if you are feeling superior (resources for learning both are in the bibliography). Switching meditation practices for a time was mentioned in the last chapter in the context of working through dry spells, but it is also a great tool for addressing attachment to attainment or spiritual materialism. If you are attached to nothingness, perhaps practice a visual form of meditation for a while. If you are attached to blissful states, practice emptiness. Counter what you desire in meditation to help you cut through the attachment.

What should be clear by now is that as we move beyond the "beginner" level of meditation, we aren't just dealing with pulling the mind back from individual thoughts. We are still doing that, as it never goes away, but at this level we are also dealing with the entire conditioned structures that give rise to the setbacks we experience. We aren't just noticing and letting go of the thought "Boy, I'm really progressing! Look at how much I meditated this week, I bet it's so much more than so-and-so." We are noticing the entire framework, the emotional need, and conditioned aspect of our psyche that all give rise to these kinds of thoughts—in this case, a need to feel superior and perhaps underlying insecurity. Beginning to see and let go of patterns on this subtler level is like taking off a pair of glasses you never knew you were wearing. You overhaul your entire emotional and perceptual framework for experiencing the world, and thus your perception of everything begins to shift on its own. Thus, you don't have to make yourself more compassionate out of a moral imperative; it just naturally arises because your own ego has quieted.

While described differently across various spiritual traditions, all include this kind of personal shift, commonly called psychological work in modern terms. This shift is how the real progress of meditation unfolds, as letting go and simplification rather than as accumulation of accomplishments. We are whittling down, not adding more, to the layers of our psyche. While the paths focused on samadhis or divine union might not initially seem to work psychologically in this way, to enter into the subtler states requires this kind of letting go. If we are weighed down with ego, we are too heavy for planes of light. We may experience some, but if we attach to them as attainments, we will just stay there and miss the greater gifts. Avoiding psychological work rather than embracing it is the next obstacle.

Practice

- - - - - - - - - -

IDENTIFYING AND RELEASING ATTACHMENT

There is nothing wrong with enjoying our meditation—as I've already stated, I think enjoyment is important! This inquiry is only for you if you believe you might be attached and it is limiting you:

- Do you have a meditation state you like to get to, a favorite feeling or experience that some part of you feels rewarded by when you experience it?

- If so, has this become an attachment—something you reach for every time and measure your meditation against?

- Unless you are training in the jhanas or a similar system in which you are consciously striving to gain control over your ability to enter such states, practice releasing this attachment. When you feel yourself reaching for this state or find you've slipped into it, imagine you are cutting a line from yourself to your reaching or the state itself within your body, and that this reaching sensation or state is floating away from you and dissolving as you cut the line.

- You can also try self-inquiry. Ask yourself, "Who or what is having this experience?" Really try to find the answer. This is often a wonderful complement to mystic meditation.

- Another option is to select a "counter form" of meditation to practice for a time, in order to release the developing attachment (see above in section for examples).

Spiritual Bypassing and Disassociation

When we use meditation or other spiritual practices as a means of avoiding looking at ourselves, we are engaging in what's come to be called "spiritual bypassing." Part of meditation's value is that within it, we come face to face with the many thoughts and emotions that repeatedly arise within us. For true growth, we need to create a bridge between our meditation and the rest of our life, noting the thoughts and emotions that frequently arise and seeking to uncover the deeper conditioned patterns that birth them. Depending on what we are dealing with, we may need counseling or mentoring, but with or without it (as seen in part II) some way of working with ourselves outside of formal meditation is considered part of the path in every spiritual tradition that encompasses meditation. When this bridge between formal meditation and the rest of life doesn't exist, practice runs the risk of simply becoming a form of escapism.

Robert Augustus Masters, author of *Spiritual Bypassing: When Spirituality Disconnects Us from What Really Matters,* puts it this way:

> When transcendence of our personal history takes precedence over intimacy with our personal history, spiritual bypassing is inevitable. To not be intimate with our past—to not be deeply and thoroughly acquainted with our conditioning and its originating factors—keeps it undigested and unintegrated and therefore very much present...[53]

His emphasis on understanding our past is especially aligned with Western Buddhism, within which many current Buddhist teachers and practitioners have brought contemporary psychology and classic Buddhist teachings together. But while other meditation traditions may not emphasize assessing our past as much, all incorporate an understanding of the conditioned mind and the idea that it is part of what a person seeks to uncover and see through in meditation. Each meditation style does this in a different way, but the bottom line is that meditation is about *personal change.*

If you are not changing in positive ways, you should consider whether your meditation has become a form of bypassing for you. For example, if you have come to it for stress management and are not finding yourself better able to handle stressful situations, get curious about what could be going on. If you came to it to help you deal with anger or become more patient and that's not happening, ask yourself why. If you are engaged in a spiritual journey and are not becoming more compassionate or ethical—foundational changes in every tradition that incorporates meditation—look at how you are relating to your meditation and path. Has it become co-opted by some other goal?

Of course, personal change doesn't always come easily; sometimes the process is quite painful and we might react to it by becoming temporarily more irritable or less compassionate. This kind of assessment isn't about one day or phase—it's about looking at yourself over time and being honest. Are you better able to relate to your life and the people in it in a grounded, calm, open, wise, and loving way? Look at your relationship to your meditation, too: do you use it as a crutch or an escape? The answer may sometimes be

---

53. Robert Augustus Masters, *Spiritual Bypassing: When Spirituality Disconnects Us from What Really Matters,* (Berkeley, CA: North Atlantic Books, 2010), 12.

yes, and that's fine for a time. When working through grief or a difficult period in life, we may need meditation to be a place of comfort and healing, which is *not* what spiritual bypassing means. It's only when we use meditation in this escapist manner *all* the time that it becomes a sign that we may be avoiding personal work we really need to do, work that in the long run will make us happier than the temporary highs of even the most bliss-filled meditation.

Bypassing tendencies might also arise because some part of us feels we cannot face a certain memory or pain. In psychological terms, this reluctance or refusal may rise to the level of disassociation, which is a response to trauma and a survival strategy—it's our mind's way of helping us survive something that seems unsurvivable. Disassociation might occur during a traumatic event or after, wherein a person experiences it as a post-traumatic response. There are lots of ways to disassociate but what they all have in common is the experience of disconnecting from the body and present awareness. Meditation can become a form of disassociation, a way of leaving the present moment and avoiding uncomfortable feelings and memories through altered states. We may have difficulty determining when this is a problem because there is healing value in the access of and rest within certain states. As with bypassing, determining whether meditation has become dissociative requires examining the progress you are making outside of meditation in your life.

Because I work with many sexual trauma survivors, I have frequently seen the subtle ways that meditation and healing practices can become dissociative. This doesn't mean an individual isn't benefiting in some way, but often they could benefit more through combining these practices with a deep body connection and working to relate to their practice differently. Take the example of Sheila, a childhood sexual abuse survivor. Abused by a neighbor over a period of years when she was between the ages of six and eight years old, Sheila lived with her alcoholic mother most of her childhood. Battling addiction herself in her twenties, Sheila was fortunate enough to end up in a good rehabilitation program and never looked back. Sober for more than two decades, she had done a lot of work to heal from her abuse by the time I met her, and she had a powerful mantra-based meditation practice through a well-known yoga spiritual organization. But she was still struggling at work and in social situations and was increasingly isolating herself from others.

She told me that her spiritual practice was the only thing she wanted to devote herself to.

Some find going into retreat or devoting oneself to a spiritual path full-time to be an empowering, healing choice (retreat is covered in more depth in the next chapter), but only as a choice, *not* a means of escape. As we talked more, Sheila began to realize how much she related to her practice as a way of avoiding the rest of her life. It was the only time she felt *safe*, which alone had been a great source of strength for her for a long time, and had gotten her through many rough patches. But now it was becoming a means of disconnecting from people and responsibilities, rather than a ground for growth. She began to notice her tendency to go "out" (as she put it) into a particular state she liked in meditation in which she had every little awareness of her body. She recognized the similarities between this and states she used to take herself into as a child in order to get through difficult days. She realized she needed to break this pattern and entered a mindfulness program for trauma survivors to help her re-orient to meditation and make some shifts in her life. She stayed on her core spiritual path and eventually returned to her mantra-based meditation practice, but felt it was now enriched by the new body presence she felt and that her practice increased her capacity for engagement with others rather than diminishing it.

With the right modality and guidance, meditation can be tremendously helpful to trauma survivors. Psychologist and Buddhist teacher Tara Brach describes how she sees the benefits of mindfulness-based meditation for trauma:

> In both Buddhist psychology and Western experiential therapy, this process of experiencing and accepting the changing stream of sensations is central to the alchemy of transformation. Emotions, a combination of physical sensations and the stories we tell ourselves, continue to cause suffering until we experience them where they live in our body. If we bring a steady attention to the immediate physical experience of an emotion, past sensations and stories linked to it that have

been locked in our body and mind are "de-repressed." Layers of historic hurt, fear or anger may begin to play themselves out in the light of awareness.[54]

In describing her work with clients, Tara notes how important it is to find a modality that creates a sense of safety and how it differs from person to person. One person might find focusing on the breath peaceful and anchoring, while for another this is triggering, where instead affirmations or mantras such as "I am safe" might be more helpful. This kind of choice and individualization are really the root of trauma sensitivity when it comes to meditation, the honoring of your needs and creation of a practice that supports your ability to face uncomfortable or painful thoughts and emotions so that you can be free of their harm when repressed. The process of choice and tailoring to your needs and comfort must be gently and compassionately paced, with no sense of forced releases or catharsis.

In fact, gentleness and compassion are good whenever these meditative tendencies are discovered. If you believe your meditation practice has become a form of egoism, bypassing, or disassociation, this is a valuable insight that can support your growth; beating yourself up over it isn't helpful and can even become its own kind of egoism or bypassing. Your insight may be a sign you need a teacher or counselor if you don't already have one, or that you need to ask them for help if you do. The issue may be something you can work through on your own, through changing your practice, or engaging in inquiry or post-meditation work. In a lifetime of meditating, most of us will cycle in and out of many of these tendencies in some way. Awareness is everything in meditation (literally!), and that you have become aware of an issue is already halfway to changing. Above all, befriend yourself, and relate to your meditation practice as a place that you come to with openness, honesty and compassion, as you do the best of friends.

- - - - - - - - - - - -

54. Tara Brach, "The Power of Radical Acceptance: Healing Trauma through the Integration of Buddhist Meditation and Psychotherapy," TaraBrach.com, https://www.tarabrach.com/articles-interviews/trauma/.

Practice

- - - - - - - - - -

COUNTERING DISASSOCIATION

- Two of the best counter practices if you feel you are disassociating in meditation are lovingkindness (*metta*) practice and somatic (body) awareness—focusing on emotional connectivity or physical connection.

- You can use the metta Practice described at the end of the first section in chapter 4, or the mindfulness of breath Practice from chapter 2. The grounding exercise from the prior Practice in this section can be helpful too.

- Consider seeking professional support to help you counter any disassociating or bypassing tendencies if they are inhibiting your ability to function well in your life, or are part of a larger trauma response.

Intellectualization and Conceptualization

There is one more meditation trap I think is important to cover, and it's one I think Westerners are particularly prone to: relating to meditation solely through the intellect or conceptualization. The Western philosophical tradition is rooted in the supremacy of thought—Descartes famously declared "I think therefore I am," a way of relating to our experience that affects the way we relate to spirituality. With so much material now available to us as well as a strong emphasis on reason and science as the primary modes of knowing, it's easy for us to *read* about nonduality, nirvikalpa samadhi, or even the kundalini rising, and thus believe we have *realized* these. Through the conceptual understanding that we believe we have, we may even replicate such experiences, *creating* them in our meditation based on their description rather than going through the meditative process within which they naturally arise.

Comprehending a description of samadhi, a jhana, St. Teresa's seventh mansion, nonduality, or da'at is not the same thing as realizing it. While intellectual study is an important part of every tradition and part of what helps us to process and integrate our meditation experiences, it can also be used as a way of blocking physical, emotional, and energetic sensations within meditation, i.e., using the intellect to separate the mind and body, whereas meditation is about experiencing the totality of the self. While so valuable in helping us assess whether we are falling into any of the meditation traps we've already covered in this chapter, personal inquiry and insight can also come to dominate us so completely that it becomes another form of repression. Mentality becomes our only mode of knowing, and through it we shut down all other aspects of ourselves. This tendency is often fear-based and can in fact be a type of disassociation—a way of dwelling on thought to avoid emotions, memories, or sensations that feel overwhelming.

The emphasis on detachment or non-attachment in most meditation traditions (especially in early stages) can lead to similar problems. We might repress our emotions or denigrate the sensations of our body in the name of *not attaching*. We might blank out in our meditation, believing that entering into a numb, disengaged state is what non-attachment means, but really all we are doing is creating one big mental wave of blankness that we then cling to like a life raft. The difference is between *letting go* versus *repressing* thoughts, emotions, and sensations. In any meditation form we train in noticing what is arising, but it's what we do once we've noticed that makes the difference. Again, it is key to examine how we are changing in our lives— are we growing more compassionate and better able to connect with others? Or are we disengaging and judging more?

Modern practitioners within inquiry and insight-based traditions can be especially prone to this trap of intellectualization. Traditionally, it is balanced with lovingkindness, compassion or devotional practices, or with service to others. When this balance isn't present, a practice can become dry—a person may be able to dissect the functioning of the mind at a very refined level but be out of touch with the rest of themselves. Of course, every form of practice has risks in isolation. Energy-based practices can be more prone to support bypassing and disassociation, devotional practices can tip into dependency or deification, and compassion practices can become martyrdom. Above all, we are most vulnerable to these traps when we separate our meditation from the rest of our life. It's common to hear "your life is your practice," but harder to live this as the truth. We want so much for our meditation practice to be the antidote for the rest of our life, but it often functions more like a mirror that shows us the truth about ourselves. The real work is what we do with this truth once we've seen it.

After reading this chapter, you may wonder if meditating is dangerous! It is rarely dangerous, but sometimes it is radical. Whatever your reason for meditating, changing is involved, which means overthrowing old ways of being. The parts of us that resist change usually do so out of fear, and in fact all of the meditation traps covered in this chapter are rooted in fear. If you feel you may have fallen into any of them, recognize fear may be at the root and be compassionate and gentle with yourself. Recognize too that you already possess the wisdom you need to change your relationship to your meditation. That this wisdom lies latent within you is taught within every meditation tradition, and ultimately uncovering all that blocks this natural wisdom and connection to spirit is the essence of every form. The process of discovering obstacles in order to see our way through them is a natural part of our growth trajectory. You have not "messed up" or even gotten off track— you have just uncovered another layer of yourself. No practice is ever wasted.

Contemplations

- Have you had experiences you consider mystic? What is the wisdom they imparted to you? Did you try to replicate the experiences and did this work? Do you feel you got attached in a way that did not serve you?

- Do you feel your intuition, ability to sense energy, or any other ability that might be considered a "siddhi" has increased through meditation? Do you feel you possess any siddhis, whether or not you feel you obtained these through meditation? Are you attentive to when you utilize these abilities? What conscious ethical boundaries do you have for yourself in regards to them and other people?

- Do you find yourself often thinking about your level of spiritual attainment? Has your attitude towards other people slipped into judgment or superiority based on your sense of attainment? If so, what practice might help you release this?

- Do you have tools or resources for working through emotions and emotional patterns outside of meditation that arise for you? Do you welcome learning of new patterns within yourself so that you may work through them and be free of them? Do you feel you have any tendencies to bypass or disassociate through your meditation? If so, what resources do you think you need to address this?

- Are you very intellectual in relation to spiritual study? Do you think you seek to create states in meditation that you have read about as "ideas"? Can you experience directly, without the medium of your conceptual mind?

NINE

RETREAT AND PILGRIMAGE

Both retreat and pilgrimage have been a big part of my own meditation path. As a lay practitioner with a busy career and family life, getting away at times to focus solely on my practice has been essential. Both retreat and pilgrimage are a valued part of most spiritual traditions. The early Christian "desert mothers and fathers" retreated in caves, as did Saint Francis of Assisi and the later monks and nuns of his Franciscan order. A long tradition of both group and solo retreat exists within yogic and Buddhist traditions, including an emphasis within some lineages on formal three-year or twelve-year solo retreats. Pilgrimage to Mecca is undertaken annually by thousands of Muslims, considered a religious duty that should be carried out once in a lifetime by any Muslim able to do so.

Retreat and pilgrimage are of course not the same thing, but they may overlap. By retreat I mean any time you remove yourself from your daily routine and activity to focus on meditation. This may involve a group retreat where you are meditating with others, or a solo retreat lasting from a day to years. The focus when on retreat is meditation practice, and everything involved in its planning revolves around supporting this. By contrast, a pilgrimage is more about where you are going—it might be to spiritual landmarks or areas, actual religious or historical sites, natural wonders of the world, or places considered to be energetically conducive to spiritual insight and power. Retreat and pilgrimage may be combined, as when a person travels from place to place and spends time meditating in each, or in a journey to a retreat center that is itself a sacred site.

Most of these kinds of retreats are spiritual in nature, but there is great value in engaging in retreat even if your meditation is not spiritually motivated. Dan Harris, news anchor and author of *10% Happier,* turned to meditation for stress management after suffering an on-air panic attack. Though initially skeptical, he experienced enough benefits through his practice to take the advice of his meditation mentor to attend a ten-day group mindfulness meditation retreat with well-known teacher Joseph Goldstein. Harris found the intensive practice and silence challenging, and after a few days felt so miserable and out of place he considered leaving. With help from his retreat mentor, he gradually began to relax into his practice, and eventually experienced "choiceless awareness," full presence in the moment without judgment or projection. This began to redefine meditation for him and helped him understand the true value of retreat:

> Having been dragged kicking and screaming into the present, I'm finally awake enough to see what I could never see in my regular life. Apparently there's no other way to get here than to engage in the tedious work of watching your breath for days. In a way, it makes sense. How do you learn a sport? You do drills. A language? Conjugate endless verbs. A musical instrument? Scales. All the misery of repetition, the horror of sitting here in this hall with these zombies suddenly seems totally worth it.[55]

Harris's chapter on his retreat experience does a great job depicting the ups and downs that can occur. After his high experience, he is frustrated when it doesn't happen again and has to work through other emotional obstacles. Used to relating to everything as a source of achievement, he finds

---

55. Dan Harris, *10% Happier Revised Edition: How I Tamed the Voice in My Head, Reduced Stress Without Losing My Edge, and Found Self-Help That Actually Works—A True Story,* (New York: Dey Street Books, 2019), 140.

it difficult *not* to relate to his meditation in the same way. Nevertheless, he realizes upon returning home that his relationship to his own mind has forever shifted. He has a new commitment and respect for meditation and its potential, as well as a deeper sense of what it means to truly let go and relax. These revelations become the foundation from which he is able to reshape how he relates to the stress and anxiety of his chosen profession.

On the other end of the retreat spectrum are the long-term solo retreats of serious contemplative practitioners. Within virtually every spiritual tradition have been men and women who chose to live in hermitage for years at a time, perhaps even for much of their lives. Because we are all so accustomed to being so connected in this day and age, the desire to live a life in seclusion can be difficult for modern practitioners to understand. Some consider it selfish or indulgent, a shirking of worldly responsibility or accountability. But within many of these traditions, engaging in such retreat is far from being considered escapist—it is viewed as a gift to others. Jetsunma Tenzin Palmo, who in 1964 became only the second Western woman to be ordained in the Vajrayana Tibetan Buddhist tradition, spent twelve years in retreat in a small Himalayan cave-cabin, three of those years in strict meditation retreat. She describes the true motivation:

> To my mind the contemplatives and the solitary meditators are like lighthouses beaming out love and compassion on to the world. Because their beams are focused they are very powerful. They become like generators—and they are extremely necessary…I got a letter from a woman who said that her son was dying of AIDS and that in the moments of her deepest depression she'd think of me up in my cave and that would give her solace. It's true of many people leading this life. I know Catholics who feel inspired that Christian contemplatives are praying for the world's sinners. What people have to remember is that meditators in caves are not doing it for themselves—they're meditating on behalf of all sentient beings.[56]

- - - - - - - - - - -

56. Vickie Mackenzie, *Cave in the Snow*, (New York: Bloomsbury, 2008), 196.

What this quote points to is that like our meditation practice, motivation is everything when it comes to retreat. Retreat can become an ego trip, a way to rack up hours or days of meditation in a competitive drive to prove we are more serious or deeper than others we know. This competitive sense can become dominated by the drive to have dramatic meditation experiences, psychic visions, or deep catharsis. In solitude there is no one around to call our bluff or point out the ways we are fooling ourselves. Conversely, with the right motivation, planning and guidance retreat can foster a rich deepening of our practice that benefits us and in turn benefits all those with whom we are linked.

Group vs. Solo Retreat

If you have never engaged in retreat, a group meditation retreat is often the best way to start. Most meditation retreats revolve around learning or deepening a particular practice, and include group meditation sessions, instructional sessions, Q & A with a qualified teacher, and sometimes individual meetings with a teacher or mentor. The entire retreat schedule is part of the experience and may include periods of silence between sessions, or group activities other than meditation. A group retreat schedule may feel restrictive at first, especially if you are independent and used to establishing your own routine. However, participating in such a schedule and not having to decide what you are doing next is part of the value of a group retreat. Think of the retreat as a container that holds you, within which you can let go of your usual concerns and focus on your own practice and growth. It is not a vacation or spa trip; going into it with relaxation as your primary motivation probably won't work. There are spas and resorts that do offer retreats that are more relaxation oriented (usually with spa and free time built in), but these will be light on true meditation instruction. It is essential to carefully contemplate what you are looking for and need so you can decide what kind of retreat you'd like and where you'd like to go for it.

Equally important is being sure that you are comfortable with the meditation modality being taught, the tradition it is from, and the teachers involved. Research all three, and also gather as much info as you can about the retreat schedule, contents, prerequisites, and location. Make sure you are comfortable with the accommodations and food offerings as well. Then start out small if possible—try a weekend retreat if this is offered. Some centers do not offer two- or three-day retreats and specialize instead in an immersion approach, offering only retreats of a week or longer, even to beginners. The idea is that it takes the average retreatant at least this long to disconnect from daily life and for a deepening in practice to occur or insight to arise. While I myself believe this is often the case and very much encourage retreats of at least a week, a week or more is not always the best starting point and not the right choice for everyone. Especially if you have struggled with depression, anxiety, or any other mental health challenges, diving straight into a longer retreat may not be the best choice for you. The rigid schedule and intensity of emotions that sometimes arise may become triggering or make you feel trapped. While good retreat leaders will know how to guide you through these feelings, unless you know them from before your retreat, you won't know going in that they are a good match for you. If you have any concerns, trying a weekend workshop might be the best first step. And if you are actively in therapy or working with a mental health practitioner, consult with them before deciding to go.

In group retreat, often the greatest gifts and the greatest challenges come from the same source—your fellow retreatants. As Dan Harris's description of his fellow retreatants as "zombies" in the earlier quote depicts, his initial feelings about them was not warm and fuzzy. By the end however, he deeply bonded with them all and felt a profound appreciation and gratitude for the time they shared together. On retreat, it is common to feel both toward your fellow practitioners. If you have not had to live in close quarters with a stranger for a while, the restlessness of your neighbor during practice, snoring of your roommate at night, or incessant questions by the talkative members of your group may drive you crazy. But assuming you are on retreat to help you deal better with your daily life, these challenges offer the perfect opportunity. By being removed from your "people," routine, and daily busyness, all of your inner reactions become magnified. The retreat is like a petri dish in which you are both the observer and the observed. Viewing whatever arises, including feelings toward your fellow retreatants as something to look at and work with can provide great opportunity for growth. You may just find lifelong friends on retreat—after all, where better to find individuals who share your values and priorities?

By contrast, solo retreats do not involve the gifts or challenges of dealing with others…instead you are dealing 100 percent with yourself. While it may seem self-evident, it certainly is not without its own challenges. Without anyone there telling you what to do or where to be, you must structure your own day and hold yourself accountable. When challenges arise—outer or inner—you work through them yourself (although it's always advisable to have a mentor on call, something covered in the next section). As with group retreat, it's very important to determine your motivation and use it to guide your decisions on where you will conduct your retreat and for how long. Make sure you choose a location in which you feel safe and supported, and start with small amounts of time. Many retreat centers offer the option of renting a room or cabin for solo retreats; this may be a great way to start.

It is also possible to do a solo retreat at home; over a weekend can work. Since part of the point is to disconnect from your usual routine, it can be challenging when all the signs of your usual life are around you, i.e., the mail, the paperwork you haven't gotten to, the closet you've been meaning to clean out (not to mention your phone, laptop, and television). That said, trying a retreat at home may be a great first-time option for you, especially if you are nervous about it for any reason. Ideally, spend the entire time in a room of your house that you don't normally reside in. A friend of mine occasionally does weekend meditation retreats in a tent in her backyard. Her spouse and children respect her space, and being as close as her backyard allows her to fit retreat into a busy work and family life without spending a lot of time or money on travel. She considers her backyard campouts her "reset" time, and although her family was initially skeptical, they have learned that it benefits everyone when she has the time and space to do it regularly.

Retreat Essentials

While the title of this section may sound like I'm about to offer a packing list, I'm not. That said, do not underestimate the importance of proper packing: if going to a retreat center, carefully read their packing suggestions, and on a solo retreat, make sure you know what you'll need and what to expect. (My best advice from experience is to study the weather, and, as I once learned the very hard way, find out if you need mosquito netting or bug repellent!). While your packing list will depend on where you are going, the essentials of a good retreat, solo or group, are more inner.

Whether you retreat at home or travel far away, a retreat is always a journey—a journey outside your usual daily routine. The purpose of retreat is to clear the decks of your mind, which allows you to discover a layer of your being that is difficult to access within the busyness of your daily life. Sometimes you might also be seeking healing or clarity on a particular life issue or striving to break through a spiritual plateau or dark night. Whatever your intentions, it's important to trust your own intuition about what you need and to take your retreat time seriously. This doesn't mean you won't enjoy your retreat time—hopefully you will—but sometimes growth is difficult; when we are alone with ourselves, all our shadows emerge. It's therefore important to walk the line between moving outside your comfort zone and feeling supported and safe.

While every retreat is different, here are some general guidelines you can adapt for your own purposes:

- **Establish spiritual support.** If you are participating in an organized group retreat, the teacher(s) and retreat leader(s) should fulfill this role. If you are on a solo retreat, establish support beforehand. Talk with a teacher or mentor about your retreat intentions and solicit their help in planning. Make sure they know when you are on retreat, and what their availability will be like should you need to touch base. Although the purpose of retreat is to practice on your own, the increased intensity of practice and solitude may trigger emotions or issues that you need help working through. Don't go into retreat expecting that you will need help but *do* make sure you have it available. Just knowing you have the option to ask for support may help you relax into your retreat and work through challenges on your own.

- **Prepare to disconnect.** Make schedules and plans and contact lists for whomever will be handling your usual responsibilities, e.g., coworkers, babysitters, spouses, house sitters. Think of everything that could possibly come up, everything they could possibly want to contact you about, and write it down. Walk through all of it with them. This isn't just instructional for them—it's for you, too. Going through this process will help you let go once you are gone. You will know you have done all you can to ensure things will run smoothly while you are away so you can simply surrender to fate. Whatever happens that you didn't predict will be taken care of without you, by someone else—and that's okay. Even if you are doing a day retreat, preparing in this way can be very helpful. Letting go of control is really one of the most important aspects of retreat. You need to create space in your mind and being, space for new understanding to arise. If you are away and your mind is cluttered with everything that might be going on at home, you won't have that space.

- **If you are in contact, make it intentional.** If you are going to be in contact with the "outside world" during your retreat, make it substantive. If all the logistics are covered beforehand, you can make any contact with work or family purposeful and/or heartfelt, focused on connecting briefly rather than re-engaging yourself with details that will only pull you back into your regular life. That said, really question how much contact you need, how much of the urge to connect might be a fear of letting go or even a way of holding yourself back from shifts that deep down you know you would like to make. Often, we are of two minds when it comes to retreat: we engage in it because we want to change, but then when confronted with change, old fears arise. The comfort of the known begins to take precedence and staying in contact with home maintains our link with whatever's familiar to us. For this reason, some group retreats do not allow or strongly discourage outside contact. If you absolutely must make contact, try to establish when that contact will be before you leave so you (and those you are communicating with) will not spend time worrying about when or how it will occur.

- **Do the same with media, email, and the like.** Be very intentional about what your mind comes into contact with during your retreat. Turn your phone and all other devices off for your retreat (except for the few times you've prescheduled to make contact, if any). Truly be alone with yourself. Even refraining from music or reading is often useful, although if you are intentional about what you listen to or read, it might also enhance your retreat, so follow your own guidance on this.

- **Establish and follow the schedule for your retreat.** If you are attending an organized group retreat, of course this part is taken care of for you. In this case, really try to embrace the schedule and release the need for control. If you are doing a solo retreat, plan beforehand what your days may look like. It's often best to plan your retreat schedule with your meditation teacher or mentor before leaving. If you practice within a tradition that embraces retreat, there will usually be a suggested routine; but if you don't have this, determine beforehand when you will meditate each day, how many times, and for how long. What other activities will you engage in (hiking, yoga, journaling, et cetera?) Because we often resist change, without a plan it's easy for a retreat to slip into vacation mode. A part of you may not want to follow through on your original intentions, but your structure and rituals are your container for your retreat—they provide the framework within which you can let go.

- **Set your retreat intentions.** Of course, all this outer planning is really just preparation for your inner work. Why are you going on retreat in the first place? Be honest with yourself about this. What is your driving force? What are you hoping for? Contemplating this before you go will help you cut through any projections or expectations you may have, freeing you up to just let things unfold once you are there. Clarify and purify your motivation.

- **Ritualize your entry into retreat.** When you leave home (or if you are retreating at home, once you start your retreat schedule for the day), do so in an intentional way. Perhaps say a blessing for your home and ask for guidance on your retreat. Express your gratitude for being able to retreat, including thanking those inwardly who are making it possible (see first bullet point!). Mark the official entry into your retreat time with intention. Within specific spiritual traditions there will often be a ritual for this, but you can create your own if not.

- **Be honest.** Once on retreat, be honest with yourself: Where is your mind really? Are you narrating your retreat to others as it occurs? Do you catch yourself daydreaming about how great you will feel at the end or worrying about what's going on at home? Years ago, when boomboxes (for those too young to remember, giant portable radios) were all the rage, I remember going to a beach filled with competing boxes playing music so loudly it wasn't possible to even hear the surf a few feet away. Thinking of home or mentally talking to others while on retreat is like bringing a boombox to the beach. Leave it!

- **Be gentle.** There are a lot of different kinds of retreats, so it's hard to give specific advice on how to handle inner challenges that may arise. This point is more personal and somewhat guided by the spiritual tradition and/or teacher you relate to. And yes, there are often challenges; we rarely shift to a new understanding without first encountering a block. Many of the challenges discussed in prior chapters—emotional sensitivity, energy bursts, attachment to states, and so on—are more likely to arise on retreat because of the intensive practice. Working your way through these is part of the value. So, if they do come up, know it's okay. Just be honest about what's arising. If it's too much for you to handle, of course reach out to your spiritual support mentor. But also entertain the possibility that you can just let it be and watch what's going on within you…it may move through on its own. Let go.

- **Ritualize your exit too.** Don't judge a retreat. Just like meditation, sometimes you can't really tell how it has affected you immediately after the fact. Big experiences and insights aren't always the point. Simply express your gratitude and prepare for your re-entry into your regular life. Set some intentions for what you'd like to take back into your life with you from retreat. Journal or make notes for yourself to help you connect with your retreat once you are back.

- **Allow time for re-entry.** You may need some transition time between your retreat and re-entry into your regular daily responsibilities. If possible, allow yourself some buffer days. You may need time to process and/or integrate, and that's all okay. It's common to feel especially sensitive to your surroundings and others after the solitude and quiet of a retreat. Or you may feel something fundamental has shifted for *you*, but life has continued as normal upon your return with little acknowledgment from others. Energetically, you may have experienced releases that your mind and body need time to adjust to as well. It's also possible you will slip right back into daily life with a new level of calm and acceptance. Above all, be gentle with yourself and (if you can) create the space to explore this sensitivity and create a bridge between your retreat and rest of your life. This is when any notes or journaling you did on retreat can be very helpful with integration; they can help create this bridge. Talking with your spiritual support person also helps.

Pilgrimage Considerations

Most of the Retreat Essentials above also apply to pilgrimages, but you have the added consideration of place. To some extent this is also true of retreat, as any location dedicated to spiritual practice is sacred ground, and the site of many retreat centers is selected according to the spiritual power available there. You might choose a pilgrimage site based on historical significance, or you might choose it for its natural beauty and spiritual power. Many classic spiritual pilgrimage locations are both, such as Mt. Kailash in Tibet, or the Camino de Santiago trail in Spain. Depending on the emphasis, however, you will want to shift your focus. For places of spiritual historical significance, you will want to find ways to connect to the pilgrims and seekers who have come before you, literally their realizations and states of awareness. For natural locations, the experience is more about opening to the energies and vibrations available from the land. Either way, the real connection is inner, not visual or based on learning facts or culture. Those may also be interesting and spur their own kind of realizations, but it's easy to slip into tourist mode if you connect too much in this way. The value of pilgrimage is inner. Phil Cousineau and Huston Smith put it this way in their book *The Art of Pilgrimage:*

> For millennia, this cry in the heart for embarking upon a meaningful journey has been answered by pilgrimage, a transformative journey to a sacred center. It calls for a journey to a holy site associated with gods, saints, or heroes, or to a natural setting imbued with spiritual power, or to a revered temple to seek counsel. To people the world over, pilgrimage is a spiritual exercise, an act of devotion to find a source of healing, or even to perform a penance. Always, it is a journey of risk and renewal. For a journey without challenge has no meaning; one without purpose has no soul.[57]

"A journey without challenge has no meaning" is one of the common sentiments about pilgrimage expressed across traditions. We *are* meant to encounter challenges on a pilgrimage, external or internal. And often we experience both: physical obstacles we may face and even the feeling that we can't go on both reflect our inner attachments or obscurations. As we work through our external challenges, we release our inner as well. Conversely, it might feel as if it happens the other way around—as we release our inner expectations, judgments, or projections (or whatever is hindering our ability to connect with the spiritual energies we seek), we discover our

- - - - - - - - - - -

57. Phil Cousineau and Huston Smith, *The Art of Pilgrimage: The Seeker's Guide to Making Travel Sacred,* (York Beach, ME: Conari Press, 2012), xxv.

external obstacles are suddenly magically cleared and new potential opens itself before us. These kinds of stories are so prevalent in pilgrimage tales that they almost form their own genre and their own kind of narrative framework from within which we experience any pilgrimage.

On one pilgrimage to spiritual sites in Japan I undertook with a friend, she became severely ill with a mysterious ailment as we traveled. She had decided to join me because she was going through a difficult divorce but did not want to talk about it on the trip; she just wanted to get away. We were visiting Buddhist temples and sacred sites throughout our journey, ascended Mount Fuji, and meditated daily. She got sicker and sicker, no matter what she did or didn't eat, and I showed no sign of illness myself, so whatever it was didn't seem contagious. We had just decided to cut our trip short when we embarked on one last walk we had intended to do, through Okunoin, a large forest cemetery with a long meandering pathway through towering trees and awe-inspiring shrines and tombs. Around one shrine we found many tiny statues, some of which were covered in children's clothing. The shrine was for children who had been born stillborn or died as babies or toddlers. As we learned this, my friend began to cry. She had given birth to a stillborn baby several years before.

Once the tears started, they wouldn't stop. We sat down in the forest and she cried for several hours. Eventually she began to talk and shared that she felt the loss of her stillborn son had marked the beginning of the end of her marriage. She and her husband had grieved differently; while she had wanted to mark their son's birthday annually in his remembrance, her husband had just wanted to move on and viewed her continued mourning as needless self-punishment. She had internalized a lot of self-blame, wondering if she could have done something differently during her pregnancy to prevent the tragedy. She and their marriage had never fully recovered. Here in the forest, she realized how much she needed to mourn the loss of her child *and* her marriage.

By the time we returned to our room that night, a remarkable thing had occurred: my friend no longer felt sick. In fact, although sad, she felt better physically than she had in months. We continued with our trip, but she now considered it not as an escape from her pain but as a container for experiencing it, alternating between mourning, reminiscing, and eventually, contemplating what it meant to move forward with her life. This kind of trajectory is not unusual on pilgrimage *or* retreat. We don't always have something so specific to process, but when we do pilgrimage in particular, it can be the perfect container for doing so, and the obstacles we encounter are often a reflection of the inner work we are doing.

Part of what triggered my friend's release was our attention to this sacred place. As we walked among the forest shrines, we both felt ourselves pulled into a deep silence. While it was somewhat uncomfortable to be surrounded by the signs of so much death, we both recognized a spiritual power there we needed to connect with. Intending to connect on this level is the most important thing you can do on pilgrimage. In many places, you may be surrounded by tourists who are more interested in getting the perfect photograph or accumulating historical facts. Of course, you can do this too, but make sure you are focused on the sensory and energetic emanations of the places you are visiting as well. How does it *feel* to you? How does it make *you* feel?

Honor too when a place does not feel right for you. Natural power places in particular each have different emanations. Some are power vortexes, others healing and womblike, and still others enhance psychic abilities and facilitate visions. Each must be approached in a different way, and staying too long in one may leave you feeling unbalanced. Make sure you are safe physically and energetically, and if you begin to feel too uncomfortable, leave. Emotional processing of the kind my friend experienced is very different from feeling energetically or physically vulnerable. Be smart about planning your trip, and about tuning into what is happening as you engage in it.

Two attitudes make all the difference when it comes to pilgrimage: *respect* and *gratitude*. Whether you are visiting a historical sacred site or a natural power spot, cultivate these two feelings toward your chosen location. Remind yourself of both often and express them out loud. In many traditions, it is expected that you will offer something to any place you visit, whether monetary or symbolic, so consider doing so. At the very least, offer your inner reverence. While this is simply good spiritual etiquette toward a place that is giving you so much, it also serves you, because focusing on your gratitude will keep you open and connected to a place on a different level than trying to capture the perfect photograph.

It's also important to remember to make inner space for peace, joy, and light—on retreat and pilgrimage. Both are opportunities to feel lighter, to let go of the often-heavy weight of everyday life. Embrace these feelings, revel in them even. While we've spent much of this and the two other chapters of part III focused on the challenges and obstacles that can arise when engaged in meditation as a path for growth, ultimately these are part of the process of shedding that which blocks us from deeper happiness. It's important not to get so embroiled in the struggle that you cannot open to the joy. Surrendering to joy is as much a part of the journey as facing down our demons. Embrace it all!

Practice

CONNECTING TO NATURE

- Depending on the location, one of the most beautiful aspects of both retreat and pilgrimage can be connecting to nature.
- Try meditating outside if this is safe and appropriate, and even making some aspect of nature your meditation focus.
- Gaze upon a flower's delicacy, focus on the sound of a running creek or wind in the trees, or revel in the warmth of the sun.
- Each of the elements have links to different energies and states of awareness in various spiritual traditions, and by connecting with one or more so deeply you can settle into a slower, ancient vibratory field and wisdom.

Contemplations

- If you have been on retreat, what were the gifts and challenges of the experience? When and what kind of retreat would you like to do in the future?
- If you have not yet been on retreat but would like to, what are your biggest fears? What is your primary goal?
- If planning a solo retreat, what is your primary intention? Go through the list of Retreat Essentials for yourself—how will you handle each?
- Have you been on a trip you consider a pilgrimage? What did you experience? Whether or not you've been on one before, where would you like to pilgrimage to and why? How can you make this happen?

PART IV
MEDITATION IN THE WORLD

My focus throughout this book has been on the practice of meditation itself and how you can deepen, personalize, troubleshoot, and motivate your practice. But as we've seen repeatedly, meditation does not exist in a vacuum—what would be the point if it did? Our experiences in and out of meditation reflect and affect each other, hopefully in positive ways. The focus in this last section of the book is more explicitly about aspects of the external world and how they relate to a practice. Most of us are taught meditation from someone, in many cases within an organization and/or ongoing teacher-student relationship. This relationship is often unique, and in chapter 10 we will explore its complexities, how it can benefit you or go wrong, how to know when to move on from a teacher or organization, and how to find one if you don't have one and would like to.

In chapter 11 we'll explore how gender and inclusivity issues affect our relationship to meditation, including exploring the sacred feminine. We often think of mind or spirit as non-gendered, but our world is very gendered, and we cannot separate our practice from this. Within this chapter we'll also explore meditation and activism—how for some meditation is a revolution of mind, uprooting conditioned patterns including cultural conditioning, and how this can become part of a larger purpose and way of being in the world. In chapter 12 we'll tie together many of the themes covered in this book and cover formal post-meditation and integration methods.

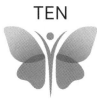

TEN

TEACHERS AND GUIDES

The relationships we have with our meditation and/or spiritual teachers can be some of the most beautiful, supportive, and empowering experiences of our lives. However, I find that the topic of spiritual teacher/student relationships has become a fraught one in recent years, as stories of scandals have broken out in virtually every major religious tradition as well as in some yoga and meditation retreat centers. Although abuses of power unfortunately occur in all kinds of organizations, it's particularly demoralizing within a spiritual context, as this realm is meant to be where our highest potential is reached and highest ethics embodied. For me, the most heartbreaking result of this is how many people have given up on the idea of having a teacher at all. While I absolutely believe that we each contain multitudes of inner wisdom that are ultimately enough to guide our own journey, it can sometimes be a tricky business to uncover this wisdom and have faith in it, which is ultimately what a good meditation or spiritual teacher helps us do. Having benefited from multiple such teachers myself, I highly value the teacher-student relationship, and wish that more meditators could benefit from one or more healthy ones.

The bottom line is that meditation of any type is meant to help us uncover our own inner wisdom and insight, and any teacher guiding us should be helping us discover this. In theory, determining a good teacher from a bad one should thus be pretty straightforward—a good teacher empowers your ability to meditate and experience the benefits and insights from it directly. These benefits and insights are yours to keep and are not dependent upon your relationship with the teacher. The teacher-student relationship is a means to an end, a tool for progress, not an end in itself rooted in dependency, fear, or disempowerment. But because we are often dealing with strong emotions and personal patterns as we delve deeper into meditation practice, it isn't always easy to see when a teacher-student relationship is unhealthy. As well, a teacher's role differs depending on your meditation motivation and spiritual tradition. Sometimes there are cultural barriers that contribute to misunderstandings between teacher and student.

Because of these complexities, in this chapter I'll first cover the different kinds of teachers we might have in the context of meditation. We'll also explore what to look for in one if you don't already have one, how to relate to one if you do, what constitutes abuse, and what to do if you believe you have been in an abusive situation. At the end, I'll briefly touch on the topic of out-of-body guides and teachers.

Selecting and productively working with a teacher is partially about knowing what it is you want and need. Again, it comes down to your motivation and recognizing that it may change over time. If your motivation when you began meditating was stress management or improved health, you may have simply needed a one-time class to get you started and now can turn to books or the occasional workshop or group retreat to get your ongoing questions answered. If you are engaging in meditation as part of counseling or therapy, your counselor or therapist may double as your meditation teacher; if they send you elsewhere for meditation instruction, they may still be your primary resource when you encounter challenges that are psychologically based. Sometimes motivation changes, so you may need a new kind of teacher to help you move forward after a time. Most of us who engage in meditation as part of a spiritual journey need guidance as we traverse the path—it is difficult to see our way through the kinds of obstacles that can arise, or to interpret our experiences. Here then are the kinds of teachers that may be useful:

- **Meditation Teacher:** These are "how-to" guides who teach us how to meditate, help us establish a routine, and support our practice. They may answer our meditation questions as they arise, help us interpret our experiences, and provide advice for working through challenges. You may only be in contact with such a teacher during a limited time course, but it's helpful to have someone you stay in contact with who you trust to guide you along the way.

- **Spiritual Mentor or Counselor:** This person may also be your meditation teacher but is counseling you in a broader way in addition to offering meditation instruction. If you are studying within a spiritual organization, there may be individuals assigned to teach classes on particular subjects, or they might provide advice on dealing with broader life issues as they arise within the context of the spiritual tradition. A spiritual mentor may also be more informal, e.g., a more experienced practitioner you respect and with whom you have a good rapport and can turn to when needed.

- **Spiritual Teacher or Guru:** This might be a spiritual authority or leader within an organization you are studying, or it could be an individual who teaches privately from their own experience. The nature of this relationship is ongoing and includes meditation as one aspect of the spiritual path. However, the depth of this relationship should evolve over time as the student "tests" whether the teacher is right for them and acts in integrity. In some traditions, there may be a devotional component to the teacher-student relationship as this trust evolves. There may also be an energetic empowerment component.

While the differences between these kinds of teachers may seem self-evident, I find that some of the issues that arise stem from a misunderstanding on the part of the student as to what they really want or need. So whether you are looking for a teacher or already have one, contemplate what it is you want and need from your teachers or guides. If you have felt up until now that you don't need a teacher or guide, it might also be helpful to revisit that feeling based on the previous list and consider whether you would benefit from one or the other, at least for a time.

Another very common pitfall in relation to a teacher of any type is forgetting that they are human. The belief and hope that meditation or a particular spiritual path will solve our problems and finally bring us the life we want can easily translate into placing the teacher on such a pedestal that it is inevitable they will fall short. We may also have projections about what inner peace or spiritual realization "should" be that have the potential to create incorrect assumptions about how a teacher should or shouldn't behave. Personally, I do not excuse any abusive behavior and therefore find it very valuable and important to see an individual as human *in addition to* whatever else they may represent. The understanding of the interplay between a teacher's spiritual power and their human self will evolve over time. It is important to remain realistic regarding people in the role of teacher or leader so that we don't fall into the traps of strict obedience or disillusion.

I myself have been fortunate to have had many good teachers of all three types and continue to do so. Continuing to be a student supports my own ability to be a better teacher. That said, many of my teachers have not been formal—my family, friends, and even my pets have been and are my teachers (perhaps especially my pets; I have often thought I could write the story of my personal growth through the eyes of each dog I've had and what they have had to teach me!). Though it may sound cliché, life and all the beings we encounter within it are our true teachers. Learning to relate to life is part of the gift of meditation. As we become more and more aware of the thoughts and emotions that arise within us and become less and less reactive, we can begin to open to what is unfolding around us, and what it is showing us about ourselves and the world in every moment. We practice this in meditation, and then we live it when we get up from our cushion and walk out into our day.

Finding a Teacher

Whether you are looking to find a meditation teacher or mentor for the first time or trying to find a new one, for the most part it is the same as finding any other teacher: research organizations and teachers that are offering what it is you are looking for, find out as much as you can about them, read things they have written if this is available, and try them out for a single class or weekend workshop if possible. See if what they are teaching and the way they communicate it resonates for you. Two people may teach the same form of meditation but communicate it differently and excel at addressing different challenges based on their own life experience. Sometimes, in fact, the similarities in life experience may be the most important factor. I was drawn to my current teacher at a time in my life when I was the busy mother of three young kids, as she herself raised three kids and is now a grandmother. She understands the challenges of balancing family life and an intensive meditation practice and can address my questions regarding it from her own personal experience. Although these kinds of personal similarities may not always be necessary, they can be helpful.

Spending time to contemplate your needs and how they may have changed is critical, and something only you can do. A woman recently recounted to me a story about recognizing her changing needs when it came to meditation instruction. She began meditating with a MBSR instructor many years ago to help with stress management. Because she had trauma in her background, she was particularly grateful that this instructor was also a therapist and trauma-sensitive. She worked with this instructor in more advanced mindfulness classes and workshops for years and experienced many benefits, going so far as to credit MBSR with helping her fully integrate and heal from her trauma; she said that she rarely if ever felt triggered or anxious anymore. However, her spiritual life had revived over the years—she had become more connected to her childhood faith of Catholicism and had joined a progressive parish in her community that aligned with her values. She even began to occasionally have spiritual visions that included Mother Mary and Jesus. Although her MBSR instructor taught MBSR primarily from a secular perspective, he was not comfortable with helping her interpret these visions, as his own spiritual proclivity was Buddhist. He often advised her to let go of these visions rather than explore them. She found herself feeling frustrated and at times even angry with him over this.

Eventually, she spoke to her new parish's priest about it. He took her visions seriously, pointed her to some Catholic resources for interpreting them, and told her he had been contemplating starting a Catholic prayer and contemplation group to focus on more meditative personal practices for those interested. He counseled her that there was no reason she could not benefit from both kinds of practices, and, based on her long positive relationship with her prior teacher, advised her to simply reframe for herself what she was getting from each practice. This helped her let go of the irritation she had been feeling, as she realized her expectations had been out of line: she could still benefit from working with her MBSR teacher without expecting him to help her sort through her Catholic faith. When a later car accident triggered some trauma in her body that she needed help dealing with, the MBSR teacher's guidance and help with her mindfulness practice continued to be of great benefit to her.

Whether it is because your needs have changed, you have moved into a new phase of life, or you have encountered new experiences or challenges in your meditation practice, you may benefit from multiple teachers over the course of your meditation lifetime. On the other hand, jumping from workshop to workshop or teacher to teacher, or changing meditation styles every time does not serve you either. This restlessness is often accompanied by a pattern of believing that each one is "the one" that will solve every problem you have. Being let down is thus inevitable as soon as some difficulty or challenge arises. Often this pattern reflects a deep need to find a savior outside the self, and the real work is to learn to move inward and trust the wisdom there, which can usually only occur for any of us if we commit to one practice for a considerable length of time and go deep with it.

Westerners have a lot of ideas about meditation and the spiritual traditions that many of the forms taught here stem from, which can lead to unrealistic expectations about what a teacher can or cannot offer. Being a highly recognized teacher within a spiritual lineage does not mean that someone understands trauma, addiction, clinical depression, or other serious physical or mental health issues. If these are part of your history, you need to be honest with any teacher you have about them and have other sources of support in your life for them. You should be able to talk honestly with any teacher you have about ways you find your meditation practice triggering and discuss ways to adapt your practice and reconcile it with your other treatments. If your concerns are dismissed, it may signal a problem. You may want to consider if you are in the right environment for yourself. The same is true in the other direction—you might encounter a therapist or doctor who discourages meditation out of a preconceived notion about it. The goal is for all the forms of support in your life to integrate and work together.

Finding a spiritual teacher may be a more esoteric process than finding a meditation teacher, although a meditation teacher-student relationship may evolve into a spiritual teacher-student one. There is a commonly repeated quote (of uncertain origin) that says "when the student is ready, the teacher

will appear" that speaks to a lot of our cultural ideas about the mystical, esoteric process of finding a teacher. Certainly, many people recount stories of a
spiritual teacher appearing in their dreams before they met in real life or of
a sudden change in plans leading to a fortuitous meeting. I have experienced
both of these myself and definitely believe that when we are experiencing
an inner longing for transformation or spiritual deepening, we will draw to
us that which we need. Really this is a kind of opening that occurs when
we acknowledge what we are longing for. Finding spiritual guidance can
also happen through much less mystic or miraculous means, too, such as the
result of an honest assessment of where we are in our lives.

However mystical and "karmic" a meeting may seem, committing to a
teacher should be a gradual process of getting to know the teacher and assessing whether they have what you need and are living in alignment with the
teachings they espouse. If you did not come to them through research, do it
once you meet them: read their books or writing, research what they have to
offer, and talk to other students. Often the latter is the most important part of
this process—talk with longtime students and see if they reflect the wisdom,
qualities, and transformation you yourself are seeking. Be wary if everyone
seems too alike or is parroting the same teachings over and over. True spiritual realization doesn't create clones.

Most of all, practice what the teacher advises and observe the results. Is it
working for you? Do you see the benefits you had hoped for? Do you sense it
is right for you? Does it resonate? It's possible you won't understand or feel
comfortable with absolutely everything a teacher advises. It's okay to bookmark certain things to assess later when you know more, as long as you aren't
forced to adopt a practice that makes you feel uncomfortable. Above all, whatever you try should resonate and benefit you in some way. If you are told "Oh,
you aren't seeing benefits because you need to attend/purchase the next level of
teachings/practices," even though the initial ones aren't doing anything for you,
consider it a red flag.

Sometimes spiritual seekers believe that this kind of pre-practice questioning and research run counter to the mystical or greater plan the universe
has for each of us, that the skeptical should instead simply trust and let go.
There is a certain amount of wisdom to this, as it's true that spiritual seeking involves faith, which by its very nature is something we cannot research

or reason our way through. I think sorting through what your spiritual path looks like partly involves acknowledging your individual patterns. If you tend to be overly cautious and analytical, then yes, maybe you need to let go a bit and trust that dream you had or fortuitous encounter. Bookmark the research for a bit and just try out the practices you are being taught and see how they affect you. If you have a pattern of jumping first and looking later that hasn't always served you, then proceed more cautiously and rationally. Spiritual realization is not a race; you can take some time to make sure a teacher is right for you. And as covered earlier, a teacher may be right for you for a certain part of your path or certain lessons. If you project onto the relationship the idea that because it began so mystically it must be a lifelong commitment (or if the teacher or organization pushes this), you may miss the next step of your path. Be open, honest, and grounded in your own wisdom.

Relating to a Spiritual Teacher

Relating to a spiritual teacher varies a lot by tradition. As you can probably tell, I am not a fan of any tradition that insists upon obedience or devotion from day one. As Eastern teachings have come into deeper contact with Western psychology, this sort of expectation has reduced considerably. The teacher-student relationship is evolving within many traditions, as an understanding of how harmful power dynamics can develop is better understood. However, devotion can also be a rich part of the teacher-student relationship once love and trust have naturally developed over time. That feeling should never be rushed.

Although it's beyond the scope of this book to really delve into the role of a spiritual leader, officiant, teacher, or guru, I think it's helpful to distinguish the different functions that often become associated with these roles. These functions differ according to the tradition or organization, and/or may be split up between multiple people in some cases:

- Ongoing meditation instruction, including how to deal with specific challenges and how to interpret meditation experiences.
- Instruction, study, and advice on the entire tradition, and all of the life aspects involved.
- Guidance on moving through the stages or levels of meditation and stages of spiritual growth, as defined by the tradition (i.e., part II of this book).

- Leader/facilitator of rituals designed to connect a student or practitioner to spirit, however that is defined within the tradition.

- Empowerments, initiations, blessings, and transmissions—these may or may not be linked to specific meditation practices (in some traditions it is required to receive the proper empowerment or transmission in order to engage in certain practices).

- Portals into states of mind a student cannot initially attain on their own. In some traditions, a teacher is able to emanate from their own meditation, i.e., a state of samadhi or level of realization, and the student may experience this through them. It becomes a reference point for the student to strive for.

- A link to the ongoing support and protection of a lineage or tradition. A lineage is usually defined as an unbroken line of teachings that have passed directly from teacher to student for generations. A student can draw upon the power of the realizations of past teachers and practitioners in the lineage, and the teacher is the link to this. Protection for a seeker may also be part of a lineage in this sense.

- The removal of karmic obstacles on an energetic level. This is considered a siddhi some teachers may have that may be used to benefit students.

Understanding the role of your teacher within the tradition in which you study is very important. Things may evolve over time, or you may engage at only some of these levels. There are of course expectations and commitments that go along with some of these levels, in terms of both financial support and practice commitments, and you should be sure you understand what these are. If you wish to study with a teacher from an Eastern tradition, these expectations and commitments may be well understood among individuals from the same culture but not as fully explained to Westerners. Ask questions! Make sure you know what is expected, that you are comfortable with it, and that it works for you. In my view, the answer, "This is how it's done in our culture" is not enough on its own. Spiritual traditions have always adapted as they have encountered new cultures, and Eastern spiritual traditions meeting Western culture is no exception. You have a right to understand and consider it a warning if you are not offered explanation when you ask.

Although the definition of the role of a spiritual teacher is different in every tradition, I think a teaching the Buddha gave on the subject is perhaps the best out there, and it applies to almost any teacher-student relationship. This teaching is called the Four Reliances:

> Rely on the teaching, not the person.
> Rely on the meaning, not the words.
> Rely on the definitive meaning, not the provisional meaning.
> Rely on the wisdom, not on consciousness.[58]

Although there are many layers to these teachings, we can understand their primary meaning pretty easily. "Rely on the teaching, not the person" means evaluate the teachings and how they benefit you—don't just take a teacher's word for it because they possess a charismatic personality, impressive credentials, or appear the way you think a spiritual teacher should appear. For that matter, neither should you rule out a teacher who isn't particularly charismatic, has no credentials, and appears differently than you would expect—spiritual wisdom and realization are not confined to a certain personality type or appearance. If the teachings feel true to you and work for you upon practice, that is more important.

"Rely on the meaning, not the words" is a message about understanding what is said for yourself, *not* simply memorizing, parroting, or obeying teachings without question. Test, contemplate, practice—make them your own. "Rely on the definitive meaning, not the provisional meaning" means to understand that some teachings may be the means to an end or stepping stones to another practice or teaching, not the final word. Thus is made a case for humility—reliance upon the provisional meaning will protect you from thinking you are further along on the path than you actually are just because you have come to understand certain teachings or had certain experiences. It is a call to keep going, keep practicing, keep questioning, and to not settle for a stopping point.

Finally is "Rely on wisdom, not on consciousness." In this context, "consciousness" refers to the conditioned mind, the knowledge we accumulate

--- --- --- --- --- --- ---

58. Dzogchen Ponlop, *Rebel Buddha: On the Road to Freedom*, (Boston: Shambhala, 2010), 165.

regarding conventional reality and the everyday world. "Wisdom" is something else entirely—the direct realization of spiritual truths, much of which cannot be put into words. Your spiritual path and your meditation practice should be empowering the development of your own inner wisdom. Over time, you should feel less and less dependent upon your teacher for this, as your own wisdom evolves. If this is happening at the same time, you will feel more and more grateful to your teacher for what they have helped you unlock within yourself. This doesn't necessarily mean that you will leave your teacher, but it does mean the relationship should evolve, perhaps becoming more based on helping you through occasional challenges and obstacles, or possibly involving less outward contact and more inner guidance. Above all, the gist is that you feel your own awakening, or your own direct connection to spirit is blossoming. Although your teacher facilitated that connection or realization, it is not dependent upon them.

Abuse

In the last decade, abuse has been uncovered in organizations of every major world religion, including in yoga and meditation centers. Abuse may be emotional, physical, or sexual impropriety. The saddest thing about abuse of this sort is that it often ends up destroying victims' relationship to their spirituality or to certain spiritual practices forever. I have known individuals who felt they could never meditate, practice yoga, or enter a church ever again because of abuse they experienced at the hands of an immoral and abusive teacher or leader. Often, these victims may have previously experienced years of benefits from these practices or a community prior to the abuse (or prior to realizing the abuse). In addition to the emotional trauma of the abuse itself, this wound to an individual's spiritual path is often the most damaging legacy.

Sometimes it is difficult to recognize abuse because spiritual growth involves discomfort, and a teacher may at times trigger discomfort in a student in order to aid their growth. Because this is a part of the usual teacher-student relationship in some traditions, students may put up with abusive behavior in the belief that it is necessary for advancement. However, there is a huge difference between hearing an uncomfortable truth or engaging in a new practice or activity that is challenging for you, and being manipulated or emotionally berated. The former results in a newfound insight or accomplishment that you now own apart from your teacher—in other words you are empowered through it—while the other leads to dependency and disempowerment. The important question to ask yourself is, therefore, "Is what I'm hearing or being asked to do when put into practice empowering me? Is it leading to insight, and greater happiness and compassion?" The answer to these questions can often be found by looking at a spiritual community. When you look at students who have been with a teacher for a long time, are they empowered and wise? Do they increasingly embody the teachings in a true way? Or do you see a power struggle—are they constantly jealous of each other, competing for attention from the teacher? Are they experiencing crises? Is there a veil of secrecy amongst a "select" group and an implication (or open statement) that you must earn your way into this select group through ever increasing financial commitments or servitude? Are your questions to senior students answered or are you told "that's just what the teacher wants" with no true information? Are you made to feel disloyal or unfaithful for asking questions at all? Is there a sense of enforced rather than earned respect toward the teacher? Are there stories that create fear around leaving the teacher or organization, e.g., that you will accumulate bad karma, or fall prey to demonic forces?

Any teacher-student relationship should be grounded in trust, not fear, and that trust should develop over time. You should feel able to ask questions, and those questions should be answered. Although at times growth requires facing uncomfortable truths about ourselves and a teacher may facilitate that, it should always feel as if it is coming from love and ultimately leave you feeling wiser and more empowered. When this support occurs, there is a deep gratitude and trust that naturally develops between teacher and student. Respect flows naturally, it is not forced. Although there is a role for devotion towards a teacher in some traditions, it is based on a trust and love that develops over time, not on blind obedience.

It can be devastating to leave a teacher or organization if you have been involved for some time. This can be the case even when there has been no abuse and you simply feel it's time to move on. Depending on what has occurred, you may need professional help to deal with the transition, and of course if the abuse rises to criminal behavior you should report it. But once all of this has been dealt with, the most important thing is for you to assess what worked for you and what didn't, and which teachings and practices benefited you and which did not. Take ownership of what worked and any wisdom gained. Try to separate the teachings and practices from the teacher. What you learned and benefited from belongs to you forever. This sorting and integration process can be difficult but can also be a very important part of moving forward. It enables you to take back your path and perhaps continue to use practices and teachings (including meditation forms) that benefit you. These are not "owned" by anyone.

Whether you study long term with a teacher or not, the most important thing is that you feel meditation is awakening wisdom within you. Within every tradition I can think of, meditation plays this role. A good teacher at any level can be of tremendous value in helping you do this. In the end, a teacher's role is to help you connect directly to your own inner peace, wisdom, power, and love. There is no greater gift than this.

Contemplations

- What kinds of teachers have you had in relation to your meditation practice, and what have you learned from each?

- Do you currently have a teacher, and if so, what category do they fall into? Are you getting what you need from this teacher? Are the practices and teachings you have received from them benefiting you? What are your challenges in working with this teacher and/or organization?

- Have you experienced or witnessed abuse of any form by a teacher? Have you processed and healed from this experience? Have you sorted through what you benefited from in relation to this teacher—what is yours to keep—versus what you want to "throw away"?

- Whether from abuse or other reasons, have you changed teachers? What has been your process in doing this? Do you feel a calling to find a new teacher now, and if so, what are your primary goals in doing so?

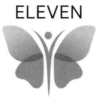

ELEVEN

THE SACRED FEMININE
AND INCLUSIVITY

The years in which Eastern teachings on meditation were migrating to the West largely coincided with the women's movement. While meditation forms exist within virtually every spiritual tradition, it is Eastern forms of meditation that have dominated in the West, through both mindfulness and yoga teachings. And while the traditions these practices came from have had some wonderful women practitioners and teachers, the majority of the historical teachers and first wave of teachers to come to the West were male. These teachings developed within patriarchal cultures where women were not allowed to participate fully in positions of religious leadership in most cases, something that is still true in most branches of all the world's largest religions today.

As more and more women from around the world have begun to engage with these traditions, a massive reexamination has occurred. This includes uncovering the histories of women mystics and exploring feminine archetypes for spiritual growth. As it relates to meditation, a lot of interesting questions have been raised: Is the spiritual path different for men and women? Is meditation different? What is the feminine within meditation? How do we bring it forth? What is the importance of women meditation mentors and teachers?

Gender or gender identification may seem completely irrelevant to meditation—after all, aren't we trying to experience a level of being that is beyond these kinds of identifications? We are, but our path to getting there is highly individual and dominated by personal history. And that personal history is especially relevant if we are moving beyond the beginner's level of meditation because the emotional patterns, challenges, and mental habits we face as we move deeper into ourselves are all shaped by our experiences in the world. These are themselves often shaped by gender or gender identification as well as by culture, race, sexual orientation, social class, and more. Finding examples and models that can address the particular challenges we face—and in some cases, the particular wounds or traumas—can be very beneficial.

Everyone can benefit from women spiritual models that reflect power and worth because historical spiritual texts often include patriarchal messages about women and feminine energy. Both are sometimes denigrated as second-class or linked to impurity. How do we separate the teachings that can benefit us from this? How do we as women in particular believe in our own ability to traverse the highest levels of a path that includes such history? How many women internalize the message that their relationship to spirit will always be secondary or must be mediated by men?

For myself, I have found great inspiration in uncovering the female mystics of all different traditions throughout history, and even entire female-based spiritual communities. From the Catholic female saints such as Saint Teresa of Avila, whose interior mansions we briefly covered in chapter 6, to the Beguines, all-women medieval communities who worshiped together and dedicated their lives to good works, Christianity has had many such models. Hinduism has produced renowned women saints such as the devotional poet Mirabai, while Sufism reveres Rabia Basri: both women emphasized divine love and had a profound impact on the male spiritual teachers of their time. A group of female visionaries lived near Isaac Luria when he was developing some of the most important teachings of Kabbalah, and greatly influenced their development.[59] Within Buddhism, Buddha's own step-mother drove him to establish the first order of nuns, and later communities of Tantrikas in the Pala period of India lived independently and shaped the development of Vajrayana Buddhism.[60] Of course there have also been countless women healers and spiritual leaders in other cultures around the world. Bringing the stories of these women out of the background of history and into the spiritual mainstream has begun to reshape our understanding of religious history, and that in turn reshapes our understanding of spirituality and contemplative practice.

Such explorations are not only important for women or those who identify as women; they are equally so for men and those with other or even no gender identifications. For meditation and spiritual practices to continue to benefit humanity, they must be liberated from the outdated and limiting cultural constraints of their time. As history is reshaped to be more inclusive, so will these practices. An exploration of the feminine and its relationship to meditation then is not meant to create a rigid constraint of a "male" path and a "female" path but instead to recognize the validity of all paths, surfacing any bias toward the masculine and integrating the feminine. Such integration opens up spiritual practice for us all.

Meditating on the Feminine

In addition to fostering more women meditation teachers and reexamining spiritual history, exploring the feminine *within* meditation can be very powerful for both men and women practitioners. Many forms of meditation incorporate symbolism or deity practice, so meditating upon those associated with the feminine can unlock aspects of our being that may not be as present in our culture. Psychologist Carl Jung first explored the power of symbolism on our unconscious and since then many healing and personal transformation methods have incorporated it. While traditional Hindu or Buddhist deity practice is often highly complex, several modern teachers have adapted feminine deity practice in ways almost any meditator can explore.

- - - - - - - - - - - -

59. See Tirzah Firestone's *The Receiving: Reclaiming Jewish Women's Wisdom* for more information on these women.

60. See Miranda Shaw's *Passionate Enlightenment: Women in Tantric* Buddhism for more information on these women.

In *Awakening Shakti: The Transformative Power of the Goddesses of Yoga,* author and yoga instructor Sally Kempton offers meditation practices for experiencing and integrating the feminine powers associated with Hindu goddesses such as Lakshmi, Kali, Durga, and Saraswati. As she notes, through the popularity of yoga, these goddesses have worked their way into pop culture, appearing on t-shirts and even in corporate marketing materials, and yet most of us do not fully understand the energies they represent. Each goddess is connected to a particular type of transformation, a power often associated with the feminine because of women's link to procreation as personal transformation is a kind of rebirth. As she puts it:

> ...[T]uning into the goddesses is a way of homing in on aspects of our own life-energy that we may never have understood or owned. Celebrating the goddesses has the potential not only to tune us to our own sacred capacities, but also to help us work with the hidden and secret forces at play in our lives. When we can do that, we can literally harness these forces for our own transformation.[61]

Meditating upon these goddesses or other symbols of the divine feminine is not a form of worship but a way of unlocking their power within us and is therefore valuable for all people of every gender. By doing so, we can challenge and gradually unlearn the still-prevalent cultural message that power is only masculine or hierarchical and therefore enable ourselves to experience power in feminine forms.

A male friend of mine I'll call David experienced directly the transformational power of such practices. David was a martial artist and had practiced an associated form of Zen meditation daily for almost thirty years. He was very disciplined in mind and body and successful in his career as an engineer. But his life was turned upside down when the company he worked for was sold and he found himself without a job at fifty years old. Entering the job market at this age, he realized his skills were out of date; what's more, a recruiter who initially sent David on interviews told him the feedback from poten-

- - - - - - - - - - -

61. Sally Kempton, *Awakening Shakti: The Transformative Power of the Goddesses of Yoga,* (Louisville, CO: Sounds True, 2012), 14–15.

tial employers was that he came across as rigid. In search of ways to change, David came upon descriptions of the goddess Kali. Feeling as if the rug had been pulled out from under him in his life, he resonated with the symbolism of destruction as preparation for change associated with Kali. He began to meditate upon Kali, including imagining himself as her and reading many different spiritual teachings about her.

It was a radical shift from his usual meditation, and the results were quite dramatic. Very quickly, David realized he did not actually want to return to his old career—something he had not been willing to face without a bit of a push. He decided to go back to school and become a therapist and has now been in successful private practice for several years. Though the path was not easy, he does not regret taking it. He credits his Kali experiences with bringing the energy of transformation and fearlessness forth in his psyche. Although David eventually returned to his Zen meditation as his primary meditation form, it was forever changed—freer and more open, aspects of mind he realized he had closed himself off from. His meditation had been a form of mental control rather than exploration, and after his time with Kali, he was able to rebirth it in addition to his career.

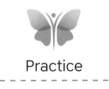

Practice

- - - - - - - - - -

EXPLORING THE FEMININE THROUGH SYMBOLS

Explore meditating on the sacred feminine through symbolism practice. I offered a brief description of this in the ancient Egypt section of chapter 9, but for this practice select a symbol that represents the feminine.

- Examples of a female symbol include Mother Mary, Green Tara, or Hindu female deities such as Lakshmi or Kali. You may also use a more generalized symbol like the moon, or a spiral (shown below)—a common symbol linked to femininity as a representation of the womb, creation, feminine energy, and fertility.

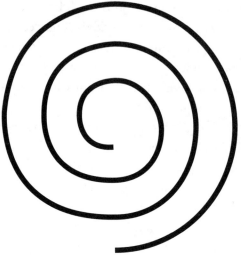

Figure 10: Spiral

- Gaze at or visualize this symbol as your primary practice for a few days (as described in chapter 9), and imagine you are absorbing its deeper significance and energy.
- Notice if you feel any shifts in your awareness during this time.

As a final note, several books in the recommended book list offer other ways to explore the feminine in meditation.

Play and Direct Experience

The fluidity David found through Kali meditation is often associated with the feminine within us that also expresses itself in lighter energies—the playful, free side of our awareness linked to direct knowing beyond the intellect, whether through intuition or direct realization of spiritual truth. In Tibetan Buddhism, this energy is associated with *dakinis*, female representations of wisdom. Within that tradition, wisdom—the kind that arises from meditation and spiritual practice as opposed to intellectual knowledge or concepts—is itself considered feminine. Dakinis often feature in stories as disguised figures who challenge an established male practitioner known for his intellectual understanding of Buddhist teachings. The dakini plays a central role in helping the practitioner move beyond conceptual understanding to direct realization.[62]

Dakini energy is as important to meditation as discipline and concentration are, especially as we progress. It is easy to relate to our practice solely as concentration training, and this may certainly benefit you if your goal is increased focus. But to access meditation's other benefits our practice needs to reflect a balance between focus and openness. Lama Tsultrim Allione describes her own discovery of this dakini principle early in her spiritual journey:

> …[]For me, spirituality is connected to a delicate, playful, spacious part of myself which closes up in militantly regimented situations. The more I try to limit my mind in outward forms, the more this subtle energy escapes like a shy young girl. It is as if I need to trust the vastness of my mind and let go, let my shoulders drop, not try to control situations, and yet not follow rampant discursive thoughts or hold on when my mind gets fixated. I think that this luminous, subtle spiritual energy is what is meant by the dakini principle. She is the key, the gate opener, and the guardian of the unconditioned primordial state which is innate in everyone.[63]

It is not that men are innately intellectual and women are innately intuitive; although we certainly may still be conditioned along these lines, it is that we as a culture have come to associate knowing only with the intellect and linear ways of being. This way of thinking has itself often been associated with patriarchy-based cultures and organizations. As we strive to understand new modes of being, we need to fully surface the often-unconscious ways we have internalized this idea about knowing. It is all too easy for our meditation practice to become fixed or intellectual. Connecting to our own innate

----

62. Lama Tsultrim Allione, *Wisdom Rising: Journey Into the Mandala of the Empowered Feminine,* (New York: Atria/Enliven Books, 2018), 111–115.

63. Lama Tsultrim Allione, *Women of Wisdom,* (Boston: Snow Lion, 2000), 28.

feminine energy and awareness is our path to balancing this, regardless of our bodily gender identification.

The concept of embodiment is also often linked to the feminine. Many spiritual paths were historically presented as journeys of transcending the body's desires, such that spirit and the divine were seen as counter to the body. In some cases, the body was even presented as impure, especially the female body. But we live in our bodies, and feminine paths have traditionally recognized this and embraced the idea of awakening in the body rather than overcoming it. Models of transcendence can fuel both spiritual bypassing and disassociation. If you are prone to either, seeking meditation forms that focus on staying fully present in your body—embodiment—will help. Recent research on how trauma affects us supports this idea that we need to stay in and work with our body to heal and change.

Practice
- - - - - - - - - - -
EMBODIMENT

- We often describe our most fulfilling meditation moments in terms of mental and emotional states, e.g., mental quiet/stillness or emotions of joy or contentment. To explore embodiment more fully, take a few minutes at the end of your meditation to deepen these experiences in your body.

- First ask yourself how you would describe the energy of your meditative state—what is its vibration, color, and qualities?

- Now imagine that this energy is spreading throughout your body and settling within it. What does it feel like to bring inner quiet to your fingers and toes? How about joy to your hips and shoulders?

- Explore embodying what you might previously have thought of as mental or emotional states.

Inclusivity and Changing the World

We but mirror the world. All the tendencies present in the outer world are to be found in the world of our body. If we could change ourselves, the tendencies in the world would also change.[64]

Mahatma Gandhi speaks here to the link between inner and outer change, which is what we strive for in meditation, whatever our motivation. If you seek stress management, meditation shows you the answer lies not in controlling your environment but in changing your own reaction to it. If you seek healing, the role of meditation is addressing the inner causes of disease, not the external. If you seek spiritual connection, meditation is about finding that inside you rather than through external worship. Whatever change you desire in your world ultimately comes from within. If we take this concept one step further and connect it with Gandhi's statement, we see that meditation is a tool for helping us change the world outside ourselves by changing inside first. While this may not be your motivation for meditating, it has this potential both spiritually and scientifically if we consider the ways meditation changes our actual brain, and from there it's easy to accept that it may even affect future generations through epigenetics.

Of the many changes occurring in the world at this time, the rise of female equality and power is certainly one of the most prevalent, and many connect this with a necessary wider shift in consciousness that needs to occur. This is not about women being in power *instead of* men but about modes of being that have been repressed (often associated with the feminine) being incorporated more into our culture and organizations of power. Really, embracing the feminine has become symbolic for overthrowing old ways of functioning that don't seem to be working anymore.

This shift is not only about acknowledging the feminine but about acknowledging all those who feel disempowered or damaged in some way, and for some meditation is a path to addressing this. Zenju Earthlyn Manuel, who self-describes herself as African-American and bisexual, defies all

---

64. Mahatma Gandhi, *The Collected Works of Mahatma Gandhi, Volume XII, April 1913 to December 1914,* (New Delhi: The Publications Division of the Ministry of Information and Broadcasting, Government of India, 1964), 158.

stereotypes for a Zen teacher. She was often counseled to drop her identifications as female, black, or bisexual as part of her "liberation." But she found her path within these identifications, and teaches that starting our practice from these kinds of very real aspects of our lives is how transformation can unfold:

> ...[I]f we were to simply walk past the fires of racism, sexism, and so on because illusions of separation exist within them, we may well be walking past one of the widest gateways to enlightenment. It is a misinterpretation to suppose that attending to the fires of our existence cannot lead us to experience the waters of peace. Profundity in fact resides in what we see in the world. Spiritual awakening arrives from our ordinary lives, our everyday struggles with each other. It may even erupt from the fear and rage that we tiptoe around. The challenges of race, sexuality, and gender are the very things that the spiritual path to awakening requires us to tend to as aspirants of peace.[65]

Many spiritual paths emphasize healing or changing the world for the better as part of practice—from the concept of *tikkun* in Judaism, to service to those less fortunate in Christianity, to karma yoga in Hinduism. Meditation can be our ally in this if we so wish. Far from removing us from the world, it enables us to engage more skillfully and compassionately within it. How this looks for each of us will be different, but seeking to incorporate the sacred feminine—whether within ourselves or through models out in the world—can be an important part of our meditation journey, not counter to it.

In meditation, we break down the walls that contain our consciousness—the perceptual and conceptual limits and biases we have placed on ourselves or inherited through conditioning. Breaking down these walls is the foundation for both individual and social change, but deciding how these two kinds of change connect in our actual lives is a personal choice that is definitely not always easy to sort through. Political dialogue and social activism can be

- - - - - - - - - - -

65. Zenju Earthlyn Manuel, *The Way of Tenderness: Awakening Through Race, Sexuality and Gender*, (New York: Wisdom Publications, 2015), 6.

deeply triggering and can themselves become endeavors of the ego that lock in our identities rather than help us release layers to see more clearly. Providing a space where we can let go of what we think we believe and release the emotions around it is another important function meditation offers in this regard. It can help us step back, reflect, see clearly what matters to us, and identify where we want to put our energy in the world.

Contemplations

- Are there any women spiritual mentors, teachers, or even authors who have influenced your path? Do you feel you fully believe in a women's ability to reach the highest levels of your chosen contemplative practice?

- What is feminine versus masculine energy to you? Do you meditate on any feminine archetypes or symbols? Do you feel both are balanced within you?

- What are your thoughts on your meditation practice in relation to helping the world? What values or causes are most important to you, and how does your meditation relate to them? Do you feel your chosen tradition is inclusive and/or how could it be more so?

TWELVE

YOUR LIFE AS PRACTICE

We began this book with the idea that meditation is practice for our lives but as we've seen, within the traditions that have probed meditation the most deeply, there is no separation between our lives and our practice. Our meditation is not an escape, and simply accumulating experiences there is not the point. When a student told the late Zen teacher Charlotte Joko Beck about a powerful meditation experience, she would reply, "Yeah that's okay, don't hold on to it. And how are you getting along with your mother?"[66]

How we're getting along with our mother, our children, our partner, our co-workers, our neighbors, and of course ourselves is really the point. Our relationships don't negate the powerful transformative experiences that can happen in meditation; meditation has magic to it wherein we may receive divine messages, float in waves of bliss, or settle into a profound peace that changes us forever. More often, however, its power to change us unfolds more quietly and slowly and may not seem linear at all. In fact, sometimes we may feel as though we are wasting our time sitting day after day. Regardless

----

66. "True Stories About Sitting Meditation from Charlotte Joko Beck, Joseph Goldstein, Sylvia Boorstein and Sharon Salzberg," Lionsroar.com, https://www.lionsroar.com /true-stories-about-sitting-meditation-from-charlotte-joko-beck-joseph-goldstein -sylvia-boorstein-and-sharon-salzberg.

of whether or not our motivation for meditating is spiritual, we need an element of faith to get us through—faith in meditation, faith in ourselves, and faith in those who have traveled the trail before us.

When we look to these meditation pioneers, we find many symbolic models for the contemplative journey. We have covered some in part II: Patanjali's yogic stages, St. Teresa's interior mansions, the ancient Egyptian *Coming Forth by Day*, and the Kabbalah's Tree of Life. And there are many other models, some of which emphasize nonlinearity—the phases of struggle, or the feeling that we're wasting our time or have taken a step backward. One idea many meditators can relate to is that of a "dark night," from the poem "Dark Night of the Soul" by the sixteenth-century mystic St. John of the Cross (coincidentally, a spiritual friend and confidante of St. Teresa). Within this poem, the dark night represents the painful periods a soul goes through on its journey to union with God. Whether you think in terms of God or not, I think we are all in relationship with our meditation practice, and the metaphor of a dark night aptly describes the more challenging days of this relationship.

In a dark night, we may feel disconnected, disillusioned, disoriented, and cast into doubt about everything we previously felt to be true. We may feel as if we've been kidding ourselves, or that we've been betrayed by the teachings or teachers we once held dear. We may feel unworthy, or simply adrift; often a dark night follows a period of great transformation and awakening, when we felt we had opened to a new level of understanding and joy. Then suddenly—perhaps triggered by an event but often not—we feel a loss of momentum, an inability to connect with our practice or the insights or peace we had previously experienced. It's important to understand that when we talk about a dark night, we are not talking about depression, PTSD, grief, or any other mental health crisis that may require professional assistance to work through. We may also want to seek help in a dark night, but really what we are talking about here in terms of a meditation practice is a loss of faith. What gets us through these phases? There are many answers, but in my experience one of the best solutions is questioning and seeking. This is why I have ended every chapter of this book with questions you should ask yourself. What has changed for you? What has changed about your practice? How have you been disappointed or disillusioned by your practice or something or someone linked to it? Usually when we probe deeply into these kinds of inquiries, we discover something we have been holding on to—

some expectations related to our meditation or life itself that has not been met. When we release this expectation, we feel a tremendous relief. We can come to our practice fresh again. Perhaps we have seen we need to change it in some way. Perhaps we ourselves have changed and can come to the practice we have been doing for years with a new perspective.

What these dark nights point to is the truth that like all our relationships, the one we have with meditations has many phases. Our growth through it is less like climbing a ladder with definitive progression, and more like traversing a spiral—we circle back over and over to the same place, but it is never exactly identical. We circle the same themes, the same experiences in our life, but each time is different, because we are different in a way we cannot see until confronting the same circumstances or feelings again.

Another helpful symbol for our relationship with our practice over the course of our life is the labyrinth—walking a labyrinth is a wonderful meditative experience in and of itself. Within a labyrinth is a definite center that we first walk toward and then away from via the same physical path, but the feeling can be dramatically different each direction. The challenge moving inward is taking each step knowing we are heading towards the center without being so fixated on that destination that we miss the step we are on. As we move away from the center and go back out into the world, the challenge is integrating the wholeness we experienced in the center with the world we find outside the labyrinth.

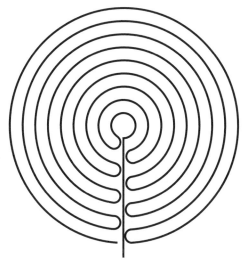

Figure 11: Labyrinth

Whatever your relationship to your meditation, it is *yours*; above all, it is a path you walk alone. While I've offered much advice in this book and pointed you to many resources that offer more, you have to trust your inner guide to know what is right for you. The point of a meditation practice is individuality, its most beautiful and challenging aspect.

Integration and Post-Meditation Support

I've talked often in this book about integration and what I've termed "post-meditation" work and wanted to offer more resources in this regard. Many meditation traditions include practices specifically designed to be done outside of formal sitting meditations in order to help bridge meditation experiences with daily life. For example, mindfulness can be practiced in any setting, and bringing our full attention to any task we undertake can help us find the present awareness that arises in sitting meditation. Mind-body modalities such as yoga, tai chi, or qi gong (originally developed to be used in combination with meditation practices) often help us integrate the energies and emotions that arise. I have found that simply setting an alarm for a few times a day and taking a few moments at those times to recenter or breathe helps me connect to my meditation and creates a bridge to it within whatever I am doing.

But when we talk about integration and post-meditation, we are also talking about working more deeply with the emotional patterns or conditioned mental constructs that we may discover in meditation or become aware of through it. These days, there are many healing and psychological models for helping us to work with these "off the cushion." Working with a psychologist or therapist may of course be beneficial, but many other kinds of counselors, coaches, energy healers, and alternative healers can help us too. Finding the right modality for yourself—and a competent and ethical practitioner—are key.

Body work can be particularly helpful; many practitioners think of meditation as solely a "mental" activity, so body work can help to unite mind and body. It might simply involve tissue massage, acupuncture, or chiropractic adjustments to help smooth energies arising in the body through meditation, or it might involve more concentrated, ongoing somatic work. There are many somatic modalities available now that all generally involve being guided through a process of connecting with sensations in the body, whether these stem from emotions, memories, or physical ailments. From there, the practitioner usually works with what is found through breath, visuals, or other activities.

On the topic of trauma sensitivity (mentioned throughout this book), some of the most helpful trauma work I have found is Somatic Experiencing by Dr. Peter Levine. He has many books and also certified others in his process. His process is also one of the foundations for trauma-sensitive yoga, and I've listed books related to both this and Dr. Levine's work in the annotated bibliography. This work is not only relevant for those who identify as trauma survivors—we all have emotions and experiences we have difficulty processing and may have repressed within ourselves. Somatic work can be a powerful way of surfacing and releasing these.

Another modality I personally practice is Lama Tsultrim Allione's "feeding your demons." Developed based on principles of *Chöd*, a traditional Tibetan Buddhist practice with shamanic aspects, this process also shares elements with Jungian psychotherapeutic methods, including active imagination. Beginning in the body, within it we bring a deep focus to how a particular memory or triggering situation feels, noticing the shape, size, color, and texture. This deep attention to our body facilitates a process of bringing this energy outside ourselves as a "demon" in order to dialog with it through proscribed questions, ultimately "feeding" it through compassion and transforming it into an ally whose wisdom we integrate back into ourselves. This practice is highly transformative and powerful in combination with meditation, and I have included the book describing it in the annotated bibliography.

Art and art therapy can be incredibly beneficial, as it offers another method for bringing unconscious aspects of our mind forward. The hand-mind link is profound, and working with modalities that empower you to draw and color may be very enlightening, even if you do not consider yourself an artist. Mandala coloring books have become all the rage and offer a way to engage with mindfulness while coloring as well. Other meditative art forms have developed, especially in relation to dance as a way of expressing and releasing trapped emotions. Explore what resonates for you, and consider it both an extension of and complement to your meditation practice.

What's important is to attend to your inner life, and as covered in part III, not relate to your meditation as a source of escape or repression, but as facilitation of an inner curiosity and openness. When we welcome what at first appears to be obstructions or challenges to our meditation in this way, we often discover through deeper work that they were not obstructions at all, but gateways to new potentials within us.

Sharing Your Practice

One of my favorite quotes about teaching meditation is this: *"I am a teacher because teaching allows me to observe the universe at work, that moment when wakefulness suddenly occurs."*[67] To me, these words capture how the real gift is bearing witness to someone else's insight and transformation. Whether we share meditation formally as a teacher or less formally as a friend or family member, it can be one of the most rewarding and inspiring things we do. But as with everything, motivation is key, and sharing with loved ones is not always so easy; after all, no one likes to be told they "need" to do something. If the motivation is to "fix" someone, it likely won't be met with openness … and the same is true if we come off as proselytizing or dogmatic.

Modeling is often the best approach when it comes to loved ones. Simply meditate, occasionally mention how your practice has benefited you, and leave it at that. Wait for the other person to ask questions and respond as best you can rather than continuously tell someone how much they could benefit. The modeling approach can be especially helpful with older kids and teenagers who do not like to be told by their parents what to do. Model and let them come to it themselves. Indeed, modeling is a great approach with anyone in your life who may be resistant: let them know you meditate, perhaps mention books and resources you like, and then just let it go. Trust that they will come to it themselves if it is right for them.

Sharing with younger kids is easier, and there are many good resources for doing so that I have included in the annotated bibliography. Kids love trying new things, but it's important to engage them at the level they are capable of. Most younger kids will do best with movement, chanting, or

- - - - - - - - - -

67. Frederick Lenz, *The Enlightenment Cycle: Twelve Talks*, (Los Angeles: Frederick P. Lenz Foundation for American Buddhism, 2002), 133.

visual meditation forms; sitting and focusing on their breath for more than a minute will often just turn them off. If they don't initially take to meditation, don't despair—again, focus on modeling. When they are older, they will remember your example and turn to it if and when the time is right.

Sharing in a wider way, by starting a meditation group, can be a wonderful way to support your own practice. I have participated and facilitated many different meditation groups over the years, and it's always amazing the additional boost this provides my own practice. However, you should not teach within your tradition unless authorized to do so if you are studying with a teacher. But do you have to teach to start a meditation group? Nope! Simply gather a group of like-minded individuals together and collectively select the practice you would like to do. Your role may be as simple as ringing a bell to signal the start and end of the meditation, or if you prefer guided methods and don't feel qualified to lead yourself, you can use recordings. Depending on the nature of the group, you can also rotate the facilitator or even the kind of meditation you do, with each person selecting a form or recorded meditation they want to introduce to everyone.

Because everyone comes to meditation with their own personal history, it's important not to lapse into the role of formal teaching unless you have been authorized to do so and received some training. Psychological or emotional issues can sometimes arise for people in these settings, and you don't want to get in over your head and mishandle a delicate situation or do someone a disservice. Additionally, many traditional texts address the "trap of mastery" or how adopting the role of teacher before you're ready can expand your ego in a way that doesn't serve you or others. But there are many other ways to share meditation without taking on the formal role of teacher.

I have personally found sharing the gifts of meditation to be a great benefit to my practice. Having to communicate my own relationship to meditation spurs me to new realizations about it, and questions from other people often trigger my own. I've also noticed that witnessing the benefits and growth others experience through their practice affirms my own faith in meditation. It is often hard to see our own growth but easier to witness in others. To witness someone blossom through meditation is a beautiful and inspiring process, and any small part you can play in this can bring you great joy. So don't be shy about sharing your practice if you feel so inspired. Just consider your audience, and what they may be most receptive to. And in all of this, know your limitations—don't take on more than you are ready for, just offer the introduction or resources and let meditation itself do the rest.

Transformation

Whether you seek to change your health, your habitual emotional reactions, your thought patterns, your relationship to spirit, or something else entirely, meditation is a tool for transformation. Its role in our transformation process is sometimes dramatic and sometimes almost invisible. When it is a regular presence in our life meditation can serve as a simple daily respite from the stress and demands of our day. At other times it may offer us strength, an opportunity to reset, empowerment, healing, metaphysical experience, grace, or awakening. It serves as both stable foundation and an ever-changing force that compels us to grow and evolve.

Nature offers us many models for transformation, and none are more fascinating—or different from each other—than the metamorphosis processes of frogs and butterflies. A frog is born as a tadpole, breathes water through gills like a fish, seemingly as far from a hopping frog as it could be. Its metamorphosis occurs step by step as a process we can easily witness. Over the course of the next several days, it develops legs, its tail shrinks, it develops lungs, and its gills disappear. Once its legs are large and strong enough, it no longer swims like a fish but leaps like a frog.

A butterfly on the other hand, undergoes a very different metamorphosis. Once a caterpillar has cocooned itself, within its hidden space it completely liquefies. The caterpillar does not transform step by step into a butterfly in the way a frog does, e.g., first growing wings, then antennae, and so on. Instead, it wholly dissolves into a liquid of imaginal cells. These cells contain the "blueprint" for a butterfly; using the fuel provided by everything its hungry caterpillar predecessor consumed, these cells gradually go about their business of transforming. The butterfly's process is closer to a rebirth than an evolution that results in a butterfly pushing its ways out of its chrysalis.

I think meditation empowers both kinds of transformation. Some changes are gradual, e.g., over time, we become less reactive and more centered. Like the tadpole, we observe ourselves day by day growing new reserves, shedding old patterns, reshaping. And other changes are more akin to what happens inside a cocoon—we experience dissolution in the light of spirit and feel wholly changed after. An old self dies and new one emerges. Certain meditations, experiences, or retreats create a before-and-after marker in our lives in this way.

While change is a natural part of life, meditation connects us directly to the power behind our capacity to change, especially once we meditate regularly and it becomes a foundation for the way we live. At a certain point, there is no distinction between our time on and off our meditation cushion. Meditation has transformed the way we interact with the world all the time, and we recognize that the power which fueled our changes was always our own, always laying latent within us as potential—just as the frog already lives in the tadpole and the butterfly in the caterpillar. It is at this point when meditation becomes more than a practice or tool; it becomes the center point from which we live, from which we become, and from which we create the world we engage with.

Contemplations

- Have you experienced a "dark night of the soul"? Did your meditation play a role in your emergence from this phase?

- How do you create a bridge between your formal meditation and your daily life? Do you engage in specific practices?

- Do you work with integration methods such as those discussed in this chapter? Somatic, artistic, or energy-based (or something else)? Are there others you would like to try?

- Have you shared your meditation practice with others? If so, how did it go?

- Are there individuals you would like to introduce meditation to? What would be the best method to help them personally connect with meditation?

- How have you changed since meditating? Have you had both "frog" and "butterfly" transformations? What additional transformations do you seek?

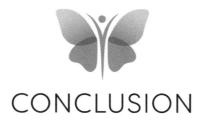

CONCLUSION

"In the beginner's mind there are many possibilities, but in the expert's there are few." We began with this Shunryu Suzuki quote ... and we'll end with it too. After everything we have covered, you might be feeling very far from the beginner's mind. Maybe it suddenly seems like there is a lot to take into consideration when meditating, and certainly this is true. But it is also true that meditation is the simplest thing in the world. In an age of experts, gadgets, and accessories, all you really need to meditate is yourself. And whatever form you are engaged in, what you seek to find is within—this is what meditation is about.

So, in the spirit of you owning whatever wisdom you gleaned from this book for yourself, let's review what's been covered in the following list. As you read through this list, engage in one final contemplative process and consider what was most helpful or intriguing to you in each chapter: What would you like to keep? And perhaps what do you feel you should throw away?

- Tips for increasing or stabilizing your meditation routine, handling a drowsy or busy mind, the most important aspects of a meditation posture, and how to relate to your meditation when life throws you curveballs.

- The way your brain changes from various kinds of meditation practice, which practices are proven to yield which benefits, as well as information on trauma-sensitivity and what science cannot yet explain about meditation and contemplative experience.

- Patanjali's eight limbs of yoga, how they interrelate, and the role meditation plays within this path, as well as the relationship between drawing inward, concentration, and the lower samadhis and the higher samadhis on the spiritual yogic path.

- The Buddhist jhanas, their role within some lineages of Buddhism, the differences between the material and immaterial jhanas, and their role in aiding the development of insight or realization.

- The role kundalini plays in the spiritual journey, and maps for meditation progress within other spiritual traditions, including Ancient Egypt, Catholicism, Kabbalah, and Sufism.

- Tips for handling intense emotions, energy bursts or sensitivity, intrusive thoughts, and dry spells in meditation, as well as guidance for when to seek outside help.

- Ways to look at mystic experience, how to process such experiences, and the kinds of traps that can arise from them, including tips for identifying and handling the development of siddhis, attachments to attainment, spiritual bypassing, disassociation, and over-intellectualization of our meditation path.

- Guidance for choosing and getting the most from meditation retreats, how to plan a solo retreat, and how to engage in a pilgrimage.

- The different types of meditation and spiritual teachers, how best to relate to a teacher, and how to identify an abusive situation.

- The role of the feminine in the context of today's meditation teachers and traditions, as well as the feminine principle within our own meditation, and inclusivity and the relationship of meditation to world service and change.

- Integration, post-meditation work, tips for sharing your practice, and the relationship of meditation and personal transformation.

Now take a deep breath. Own what is useful to you—and let go of the rest! Trust yourself. When in doubt, keep it simple. Discover the freshness, purity, and innocence of relating to meditation as a beginner—no preconceptions, no judgments, and no experience of past struggle—the beginner's mind.

> *May you discover your own inner wisdom, connection to spirit, tranquility and joy through meditation, and may it sustain you always.*

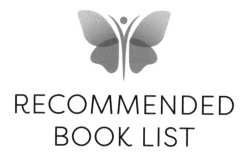

RECOMMENDED
BOOK LIST

This list is arranged by book part and is also my annotated bibliography. All books quoted are included here in addition to many others I recommend. Many of these books could go in multiple sections; in those cases, I have listed them in the section they were quoted or referenced within. At the start of each part, I have listed the topics of that section as a reminder.

Part I: Practice for Life
*Benefits of meditating, meditation
research, and common challenges*

Begley, Sharon. *Train Your Mind, Change Your Brain: How a New Science Reveals Our Extraordinary Potential to Transform Ourselves.* New York: Ballantine, 2008. Overview of latest research supporting the neuroplasticity of our brain, including how meditation impacts the brain.

Chödrön, Pema. *Start Where You Are.* Boulder, CO: Shambhala Publications, 1994. Guidance for working with challenging emotions both within and outside of meditation, including through mindfulness and *tonglen* (compassion practice).

———. *When Things Fall Apart: Heart Advice for Difficult Times.* Boulder, CO: Shambhala Publications, 2000. Buddhist and compassion meditation teachings from a Western Buddhist nun, with particular emphasis on challenging life phases.

Gunaratana, Bhante Henepola. *Mindfulness in Plain English: Twentieth Anniversary Edition.* Somerville, MA: Wisdom Publications, 2011. Classic book on traditional mindfulness meditation, including tips for handling many different challenges as taught within that tradition.

Hanson, Rick. *Buddha's Brain: The Practical Neuroscience of Happiness, Love, and Wisdom.* Oakland, CA: New Harbinger Publications, 2009. Overview of how Buddhism-based mindfulness and compassion practices affect the brain. Includes practice suggestions on how one may realize these benefits.

Johnson, Will. *The Posture of Meditation: A Practical Manual for Meditators of All Positions.* Boulder, CO: Shambhala Publications, 1996. An exploration of the body and meditation postures relevant to practitioners of any tradition.

Kabat-Zinn, Jon, and Richard J. Davidson. *The Mind's Own Physician: A Scientific Dialogue with the Dalai Lama on the Healing Power of Meditation.* Oakland, CA: New Harbinger Publications, 2013. Transcript of a conference held with the Dalai Lama and scientists from many different fields on the value of meditation and research into how it affects the brain and body.

Newberg, Andrew. *Why God Won't Go Away: Brain Science and the Biology of Belief.* New York: Ballantine, 2008. Explores research about how mystic experiences are reflected in the brain, including what science currently can and cannot explain.

Salzberg, Sharon. *Real Happiness: The Power of Meditation, a 28-Day Program.* New York: Workman Publishing Company, 2010. Classic from a co-founder of the Insight Meditation Society.

Suzuki, Shunryu. *Zen Mind, Beginner's Mind: Informal Talks on Zen Meditation and Practice.* Boulder, CO: Shambhala Press, 2011. Classic talks from a great Zen master on meditation within this tradition.

Treleaven, David A. *Trauma-Sensitive Mindfulness: Practices for Safe and Transformative Healing.* New York: W.W. Norton & Co., 2018. Comprehensive coverage of how to adapt mindfulness meditation for trauma-sensitivity; geared towards therapists and teachers, but relevant to practitioners too.

Part II: Meditation for the Spiritual Seeker
Patanjali's eight limbs of yoga, the Buddhist jhanas, kundalini and chakras, other religions' approaches to meditation and the spiritual journey

Boorstein, Sylvia. *Happiness Is an Inside Job.* New York: Ballantine, 2008. Teachings on the connections between mindfulness and lovingkindness practice.

Brasington, Leigh. *Right Concentration: A Practical Guide to the Jhanas.* Boulder, CO: Shambhala Press, 2015. Very accessible how-to guide to the jhanas based on retreats the author leads.

Dale, Cyndi. *Llewellyn's Complete Book of Chakras: Your Definitive Source of Energy Center Knowledge for Health, Happiness, and Spiritual Evolution.* Woodbury, MN: Llewellyn Publications, 2015. An encyclopedic guide to the chakras from many different perspectives.

Ellis, Normandie. *Awakening Osiris: A New Translation of the Egyptian Book of the Dead.* Newburyport, MA: Phanes Press, 2009. Poetic presentation of the *Egyptian Book of the Dead* as a spiritual guide for the living.

Erickson, Lisa. *Chakra Empowerment for Women: Self-Guided Techniques for Healing Trauma, Owning Your Power and Finding Overall Wellness.* Woodbury, MN: Llewellyn Publications, 2019. My own book on women's energetics techniques, including how women may want to work differently with their chakra system.

Firestone, Tirzah. *The Receiving: Reclaiming Jewish Women's Wisdom.* San Francisco: HarperOne, 2009. Kabbalah from a women's perspective, including stories of historical kabbalistic women.

Gangaji. *The Diamond in Your Pocket.* Seattle: Amazon Digital Services, 2004. Teachings in self-inquiry from this Western woman teacher within Advaita Vedanta, the tradition of Ramana Maharshi.

Gunaratana, Bhante Henepola. *Beyond Mindfulness in Plain English: An Introductory Guide to Deeper States of Meditation.* Somerville, MA: Wisdom Publications, 2009. Classic teachings on the jhanas from this mindfulness teacher's perspective.

Isherwood, Christopher, and Swami Prabhavananda. *How to Know God: The Yoga Aphorisms of Patanjali.* Los Angeles: Vedanta Press, 1950. Classic translation and commentary on Patanjali's *Yoga Sutras.*

Iyengar, B.K.S. *Light on the Yoga Sutras of Patanjali.* New York: Thorson's, 1994. Well-known twentieth-century yoga teacher's commentary on Patanjali's *Yoga Sutras.*

Kaplan, Aryan. *Meditation and Kabbalah.* Newburyport, MA: Weiser Books, 1986. Still considered a classic, one of the first books to explore contemplative practices within Kabbalah as relevant to modern seekers.

Khalsa, Gurmukh Kaur. *Kundalini Rising: Exploring the Energy of Awakening.* Seattle: Amazon Digital Services, 2007. A collection of essays from experts in many different scientific and spiritual fields on various aspects of kundalini.

Khema, Ayya. *Visible Here and Now: The Buddhist Teachings on the Rewards of Spiritual Practice.* Boulder, CO: Shambhala Press, 2001. Teachings on the jhanas from this woman Theravadan Buddhist teacher.

Kugle, Scott. *Sufi Meditation and Contemplation.* Amherst, MA: Omega Publications, 2012. Translations and commentary of the three main classic texts on Sufi meditation.

Lenz, Frederick. *Surfing the Himalayas: A Spiritual Adventure.* Boulder, CO: Living Buddha Press, 2018. A playful and innovative presentation of meditation teachings in a contemporary setting.

Maharshi, Ramana. *Who Am I?: The Teachings of Bhagavan Sri Ramana Maharshi.* Tamil, India: Sri Ramanasramam, 2008. Transcripts of teachings from this Advaita/inquiry master.

Merton, Thomas, and Sue Monk Kidd. *New Seeds of Contemplation.* New York: New Directions, 2007. Classic text on Christian contemplative practices.

Nikhilananda, Swami. *The Gospel of Sri Ramakrishna.* New York, New York: Ramakrishna-Vivekananda Center of New York, 1942. Transcriptions of teachings by this nineteenth-century sage, considered one of the greatest in India's history—best read in the context of the time.

Ponlop, Dzogchen. *Rebel Buddha: On the Road to Freedom.* Boulder, CO: Shambhala 2010. Presentation of Buddhist teachings from a contemporary Western perspective.

Saint Anthony the Great, Henry L. Carrigan (editor). *The Wisdom of the Desert Fathers and Mothers.* Brewster, MA: Paraclete Press, 2011. Stories and teachings of the early Christians who went into ascetic, solitary practice in the desert and caves.

Satchidnananda, Swami. *The Yoga Sutras of Patanjali: Commentary on the Raja Yoga Sutras.* Santa Monica, CA: Integral Yoga Publications, 2012. Another well-known twentieth-century yoga and meditation teacher's commentary on Patanjali's *Yoga Sutras.*

Starr, Mirabai, and St. Teresa of Avila. *The Interior Castle.* New York: Riverhead Books, 2004. A beautiful translation and commentary on this classic.

Yogananda, Paramahansa. *Autobiography of a Yogi.* Los Angeles: Self-Realization Fellowship, 2014. Classic autobiography by this famous twentieth-century spiritual teacher, one of the first to travel to the West.

Part III: The Path
Subtler challenges, common traps, retreat and pilgrimage

Allione, Lama Tsultrim. *Women of Wisdom.* Ithaca, NY: Snow Lion, 2000. Biographies of six different historic Tibetan Buddhist women teachers and practitioners, along with experts from the author's own life story in the preface.

Brach, Tara. *Radical Acceptance: Embracing Your Life with the Heart of a Buddha.* New York: Bantam, 2004. A book on transforming feelings of unworthiness (including from trauma) by a psychotherapist and mindfulness teacher.

Cousineau, Phil, and Huston Smith. *The Art of Pilgrimage: The Seeker's Guide to Making Travel Sacred.* Newburyport, MA: Conari Press, 2012. How to turn travel into a sacred pilgrimage.

Harris, Dan. *10% Happier (revised edition): How I Tamed the Voice in My Head, Reduced Stress Without Losing My Edge, and Found Self-Help That Actually Works—A True Story.* New York: Dey Street Books, 2019. Entertaining and informative tale of this TV anchor's foray into meditation and group retreat.

James, William. *Varieties of Religious Experience.* New York: Cosimo Classics, 2004 (originally published 1902, Longmans, Green & Co). Dense but fascinating exploration of mystic experience from this nineteenth-century philosopher/social scientist.

Kornfield, Jack. *After the Ecstasy, the Laundry: How the Heart Grows Wise on the Spiritual Path.* New York: Bantam, 2000. Guidance from a well-known meditation teacher on handling the challenges of the spiritual journey.

Mackenzie, Vickie. *Cave in the Snow: A Western Woman's Quest for Enlightenment.* New York: Bloomsbury, 2008. Story of Tenzim Palmo's twelve-year cave retreat. She is one of the first Western woman to have been ordained as a Tibetan Buddhist nun.

Masters, Robert Augustus. *Spiritual Bypassing: When Spirituality Disconnects Us from What Really Matters.* Berkeley, CA: North Atlantic Books, 2010. How to recognize and correct spiritual bypassing from a therapist's perspective.

Mu. *Walking the Advanced Path: Revelations and Reminders on the Direct Path of Awakening.* Seattle, WA: CreateSpace Independent Publishing, 2016. Non-sectarian guidance for navigating advanced meditative states and spiritual paths with wisdom and clarity.

Trungpa, Chögyam. *Cutting Through Spiritual Materialism.* Boulder, CO: Shambhala, 2010. Talks from a Buddhist perspective on how our ego can subtly co-opt our spiritual path and advice for cutting through it.

Part IV: Meditation in the World

Spiritual teachers, the sacred feminine, inclusivity and activism,
integration and post-meditation practices, resources for kids

Allione, Lama Tsultrim. *Feeding Your Demons: Ancient Wisdom for Resolving Inner Conflict.* New York: Little, Brown and Co., 2008. Self-guided contemplative practice for working with difficult emotions, adapted from the Tibetan Buddhist practice of Chöd.

————. *Wisdom Rising: Journey into the Mandala of the Empowered Feminine.* New York: Atria/Enliven Books, 2018. Exploration of the sacred feminine including meditations, and psychological and art practices that employ Tibetan Buddhism's five dakini family teachings.

Cameron, Julia. *The Artist's Way: 25ᵗʰ Anniversary Edition.* New York: Tarcher Perigree, 2016. Methods for working with creativity as a means to self-discovery for anyone—not only artists.

Emerson, David. *Overcoming Trauma Through Yoga: Reclaiming Your Body.* Berkeley, CA: North Atlantic Books, 2012. Based on scientific research, details a pioneering program on adapting physical yoga practice for trauma sensitivity.

Haas, Michaela. *Dakini Power: Twelve Extraordinary Women Shaping the Transmission of Tibetan Buddhism in the West.* Ithaca, NY: Snow Lion, 2013. In-depth interviews and life stories of twelve high level women practitioners within Tibetan Buddhism.

Hanh, Thich Nhat. *Planting Seeds: Practicing Mindfulness with Children.* Berkeley, CA: Parallax Press, 2011. Guided meditations for children as well as advice for introducing them to meditation.

Kempton, Sally. *Awakening Shakti: The Transformative Power of the Goddesses of Yoga.* Louisville, CO: SoundsTrue, 2012. Meditations for connecting to Hindu goddesses.

Levine, Peter. *In an Unspoken Voice: How the Body Releases Trauma and Restores Goodness.* Berkeley, CA: North Atlantic Books, 2010. How trauma affects the body and somatic methods for working with it.

Manuel, Zenju Earthlyn. *The Way of Tenderness: Awakening Through Race, Sexuality and Gender.* Somerville, MA: Wisdom Publications, 2015.

Rethinking identify and social engagement within the context of Buddhism and spirituality in general.

Shaw, Miranda. *Passionate Enlightenment*. Princeton, NJ: Princeton University Press, 1994. History of Tantric Buddhism and especially the role of women Tantrikas.

Snel, Eline. *Sitting Still Like a Frog: Mindfulness Exercises for Kids (and Their Parents)*. Boulder, CO: Shambhala, 2013. Eleven guided meditations with CD for ages five through twelve.

Starr, Mirabai. *Wild Mercy: Living the Fierce and Tender Wisdom of the Women Mystics*. Boulder, CO: Sounds True, 2019. Part spiritual memoir and part stories from the lives of women mystics across multiple traditions.

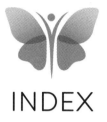

INDEX

To Write to the Author

If you wish to contact the author or would like more information about this book, please write to the author in care of Llewellyn Worldwide Ltd. and we will forward your request. Both the author and publisher appreciate hearing from you and learning of your enjoyment of this book and how it has helped you. Llewellyn Worldwide Ltd. cannot guarantee that every letter written to the author can be answered, but all will be forwarded. Please write to:

Lisa Erickson
℅ Llewellyn Worldwide
2143 Wooddale Drive
Woodbury, MN 55125-2989

Please enclose a self-addressed stamped envelope for reply,
or $1.00 to cover costs. If outside the U.S.A., enclose
an international postal reply coupon.

Many of Llewellyn's authors have websites with additional information and resources. For more information, please visit our website at http://www.llewellyn.com.